COVID

AND COMING CHAOS

Published by Southwest Radio Church of the Air

Printed in United States of America

ISBN # 979-8-89298-465-2

COVID

AND COMING CHAOS

LOU & ELIZABETH
CAVERLY

This book is dedicated to our loving parents
who first guided us to know our
Precious Savior, Jesus Christ:
Luther and Adeline Caverly and
Charles and Margaret Cuppett.

CONTENTS

BOOK TWO
NWO CHAOS COMMENCES

Introduction

As independent Christian radio broadcasters (called by God, we earnestly believe, in 2003) we began "The Divided Kingdom." This "watchman" radio ministry is patterned after the commandments of Almighty God in Ezekiel, chapter 33. Listen to our archived programs at Divided-KingdomRadio.com. Hear us at WWCR.com, Thursdays at 8:00 p.m. (Eastern Time) and their shortwave radio, 4.840 MHz.

The format of our book includes one or both of our signatures at the end of a chapter. These chapters quote extensively from various news sources and publications. Many of the chapters were originally broadcast as "radio monologues" or "radio dialogues" written and delivered by either Lou Caverly or Elizabeth Cuppett-Caverly, or both. For this reason, chapters give credit at each one's end to Lou or Elizabeth.

For example, Lou Caverly's "Bleeding Kansas" essay delineated not only present-day abortion law concerns, but also gave fascinating historical Civil War era precedents.

It is our earnest mission to continue to warn God's Remnant of present and coming dangers, many deliberately obfuscated or totally covered up by the mainstream media, as well as always to witness to the forgiveness of any and all sins, available through remorse and acceptance of the eternal salvation of Jesus Christ alone.

BOOK ONE

2020—COVID COMES

"Yes, the COVID pandemic grabbed us around our throats. None of us ordinary people ever saw it coming! Without warning, our world was turned completely upside down. How did this chaos originate? The title of this book is *COVID and Coming Chaos ...*"

CHAPTER ONE

Are We Living in "God's Judgment" or "End-Times"?

Picture this: a true story told on air by the late Dr. Carl Sanders, who helped G.E. and the government develop an early microchip. He was dying of colon cancer in 1990, and he repented at that time, giving his life over to Jesus Christ. Becoming an evangelist, he and his wife Ruby traveled all over the United States. Ruby's special ministry was to encourage women not to abort their babies. Carl told on our program, "The Divided Kingdom," how he and Ruby returned to hold a meeting in a church they had visited three years earlier. A young woman pianist, towing along a beautiful little boy toddler, rushed up to them. She explained that he would have been aborted the next day, had she not heard Ruby's witness.

Picture also a second image Carl described: God Almighty raising a woman from the dead. It happened through earnest group prayer during one of his out-of-the-country revival meetings. This is not so different from the true story of Betty Maltz, told by the late author Catherine Marshall. Betty died from a ruptured appendix. She had been dead more than a few hours. Her pastor father was enroute to see her at the hospital when his wife got the call that Betty had passed on. Yet when he reached the hospital, he found Betty coming back to life! Betty, herself, later recounted that, as consciousness returned, she saw beautiful individual letters glimmering in light from the hospital window: the words of John 14:6— "I am the way, the truth, and the life."

We find ourselves suddenly in unprecedented years of turmoil and threat. More than ever, we all need the true witness of Christians like Carl Sanders and Betty Maltz. Yes, Jesus is real. He is our Savior. God the Father, too, is real. His judgment on evil is just as bona fide as His long-suffering love and patience.

Though God's scripture forbids such practices, numerous churches admired and supported the LGBTQ rainbow flag that flew over the Biden White House in "Pride Month," June 2023. Hanging to the left and right of this rainbow travesty were two subservient American flags. If you belong to such a church, you need to see a shocking discovery!

It is a desolate Middle East desert scene. Once in a "Call to Decision" radio interview, archaeologist Jonathan Gray described what he witnessed in the area of Sodom and Gomorrah. Gray actually validated the truth of the biblical account of God's wrath coming over the cities of the plain. The archaeologist was able to pick up and hold in his hand "hardened" golf-ball sized spheres. These were remnants of the historical "fire and brimstone."

Is it possible COVID's sudden pandemic appearance, and subsequent enormous number of COVID post-vaccine deaths are indicative of God's falling judgment on His unrepentant Church House? In support of this possibility, Dr. Carl Sanders told another sobering story:

It happened on an ordinary street in the Midwest of America. The Evangelical Lutheran Church of America was holding a special convention. They had to make a decision on a very important matter. ELCA convention delegates were, indeed, getting ready to turn Christendom upside down! "You see," said Carl, "They voted affirmatively to ordain homosexual pastors." Carl had a deep radio voice, its timbre very reminiscent of the singer Burl Ives. In that sonorous voice, Carl finished his story, "A tornado had just moved down the street of that town. Just after the ELCA vote, *the tornado turned around and came back down the street. ... As the ELCA celebrated their great triumph,* ***severe lightning struck the church!"***

Our Heavenly Father despises other abominations, too, like injecting tiny children with bioweapon "vaccines." So, here is the next picture for you to view: An AP headline, July 20, 2023, read: "Tornado damages

Pfizer plant in NC as scorching heat, floods sock other parts of US." That AP article said: "Parts of roofs were ripped open atop its massive buildings. 'The Pfizer plant stores large quantities of medicine that were tossed about,' said Nash County Sheriff Keith Stone, adding, 'I've got reports of 50,000 pallets of medicine that are strewn across the facility and damaged through the rain and the wind.'" One health plan pharmaceutical director said the damage "will likely lead to long-term shortages while Pfizer works to either move production to other sites or rebuilds." This EF3 tornado with wind speeds up to 150 mph temporarily closed a stretch of Interstate 95 in both directions in North Carolina, causing miles of congested traffic.

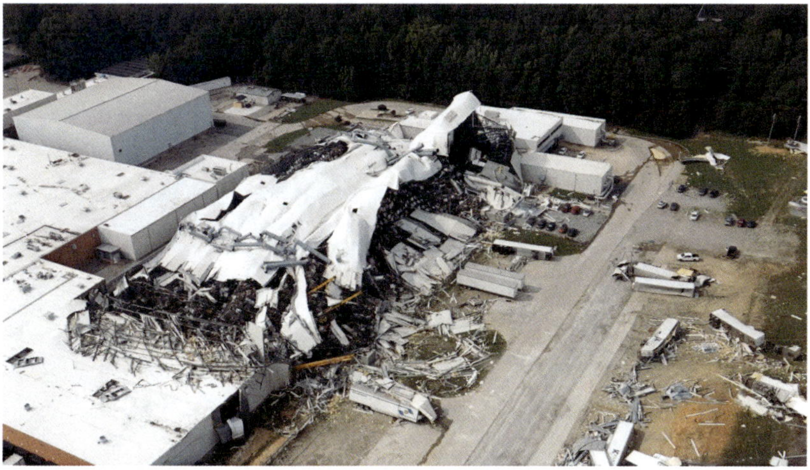

One key purpose of this book is to warn about the globalist world depopulation mindset and plan, as delineated by the Gates Foundation, the Club of Rome, the World Economic Forum, and others. Many of these leading globalist figures have openly stated to the world their approval of quickly moving this homicidal agenda forward.

Hence, this 2020–2022 scene. It moves sharply into focus in front of our dumbstruck eyes. Look carefully: ***People in lockdown in their homes. Persons wearing masks on the street. Hapless COVID victims hooked to hospital ventilators ... This is COVID Becoming Chaos.***

(As with an old-time Viewmaster) we move the dial forward two years to the hellishly hot summer of 2023 ... We are now walking down the beach to see a model home, an exhibition is called "A Ramshackle, Rotting House." This so-called People's House of America sits on sand that is shifting. In June 2023, Pride Month, this key Power Seat flies the rainbow LGBTQ flag above its front door, possibly facilitating any drag queens who want to assemble on nearby streets. They can, perhaps, entertain gathering groups of families and children as they wear tiny thongs and do "splits" (as did one drag queen star in Caroline County, Maryland's Memorial Day 2023 "Pride Celebration").

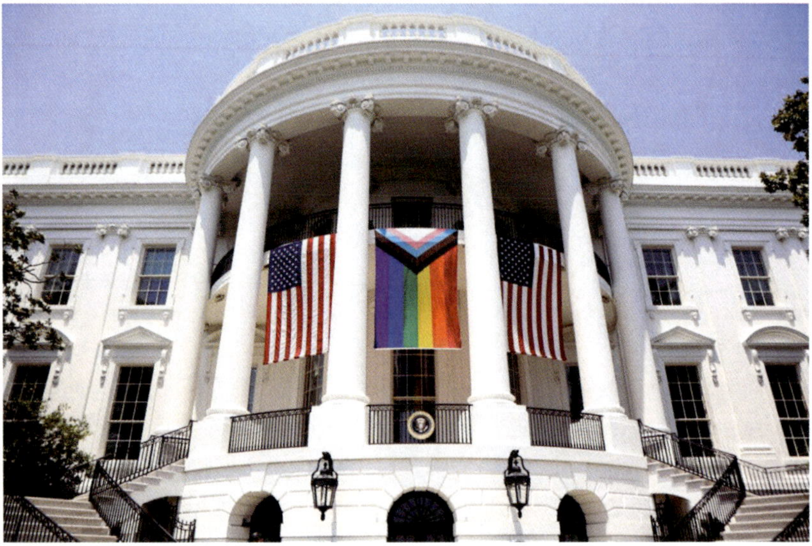

Fierce gales are howling. Fires of judgment may be edging closer. More than five hundred fires in Canada and their smoke drifting practically all over America! Soon after, radical Islam riots and burns all over France!

From Ezekiel 33 onward, God recruited prophetic watchmen to warn His people: "Visions" of Habakkuk 2:2 "written on stones" so "people could run." In *The Harbinger,* modern-day watchman Jonathan Cahn documents spiritual, historical parallels between ancient arrogant Israel and unrepentant post-9/11 America.

When the Twin Towers fell, "old boy" American political leaders had not remorse, but excessive "bravado." Both Speaker of the House

Tom Dashiell and VP candidate John Edwards publicly quoted Isaiah 9:10. [***"The bricks are fallen down, but we will build with hewn stone."***] Terrified by the New York attacks, Americans rushed to churches ... briefly. But by early 2002, many were drifting back to their comfortable lifestyles without any strong conviction for the need to repent.

Years later, these Isaiah 9:10–11-type bragging slogans once again returned. [**"Pride goes before America's fall"?**] Trump and his Maga hat followers boomed out, ***"Make America Great Again!"*** The Incredible Hulk-hubris was the real star at the huge Tulsa political gathering. [***These Tulsa attendees certainly didn't need to wear masks, or do any type of social distancing ... Weeks after, Tulsa attendee and popular politician Herman Cain suddenly sickened with COVID and died.***]

Real courage is different from hubris. President Donald J. Trump's televised brief farewell words to all of us disappointingly never mentioned ***a stolen 2020 election.*** Do these words alarm you? ***Dominion Voting Systems, January 6, jailed protesters coup against the Constitution?*** In 2023, the Biden "Rainbow Administration" still weakly reiterates the same arrogant echo of Isaiah 9:10–11. This feeble Biden and Company boast of a barely whispered "Build Back Better!" no longer convinces even those severely brainwashed.

Isaiah 9:10 states, "The sycomores are cut down, but we will change them into cedars." Another "America of today" parallel exists. Jonathan Cahn describes a tree that perished near Ground Zero in the 9/11 Twin Towers attack. It, too, was a type of sycamore (English). A new tree called "America's Promise" was eagerly planted. This oxymoronically named tree, sadly, soon died. A bad omen? ... Could this "national" tree's demise have prefigured what was to come—thousands, perhaps millions, of Americans killed by bioweapon shots in 2020–2025 and onward?

By VAERS system count, a year or so ago, 27,000 Americans perished through COVID injections. However, reputable scientists conclude only 1 percent of fatalities is reported by the VAERS system. This would indicate a possible 2,700,000 American people died by injection of the COVID vaccines. Still no repentance! America leads the world in accepting and proliferating the gravest of sins against God and His spiritual laws.

In Jonathan Cahn's book, *The Return of the Gods,* he describes ancient pagan gods and goddesses (including Baal, Molech, and Ishtar), and their present-day "return." Cahn believes these undoubted demons of Satan (disguised in mythological god and goddess roles) have been summoned. They have been called to return through portals opened by the American people's accumulating iniquities and abominations.

The year 1967 brings us another shocking picture for you to muse upon: an amazing synchronicity. As background, *The Return of the Gods* tells us the month of Tammuz was the time that the powerful goddess mourned the lover she had banished to the land of the dead. Cahn says of Tammuz (page 171), "It was the month when the two gods were separated from each other. For the goddess, it was the month of unfulfilled longings, unanswered passions, and desires denied."

Next, our Viewmaster's antique dial moves to New York City, in front of the Stonewall Inn, June 27, 1967. There, a groundbreaking riot takes place between homosexuals and police. This momentous event will change America's morality forever. This violent Stonewall revolt happens in the ancient calendar's month of Tammuz. As *The Return of the Gods* explains, June 26, 1967, the very day Deputy Police Inspector Seymour Pine obtains the search warrant for the inn (sealing its explosive fate) is the tenth of Tammuz. Stonewall's wild chaos will involve both male prostitutes and some women. NYC police run in terror and barricade themselves inside the Stonewall Inn.

Years later, a follow-up portrait comes slowly into focus. Two men are looking at each other lovingly and holding hands. The numerology pattern recurs! Yes, strikingly, that same ancient "tenth of Tammuz" is June 26, 2003. This is the day on which the Supreme Court ruled homosexuality is now legal all over America. Could this Tammuz 10 "spell" have been aided by other demonic entities, such as Baphomet, the bisexual Satan-goat representation? Did this "ancient spell" end here in 2003?

No, it did not. Sadly, the next picture we must behold is that of a man and wife having their wedding rings forced off and taken from them. The Defense of Marriage Act was shockingly overturned by the

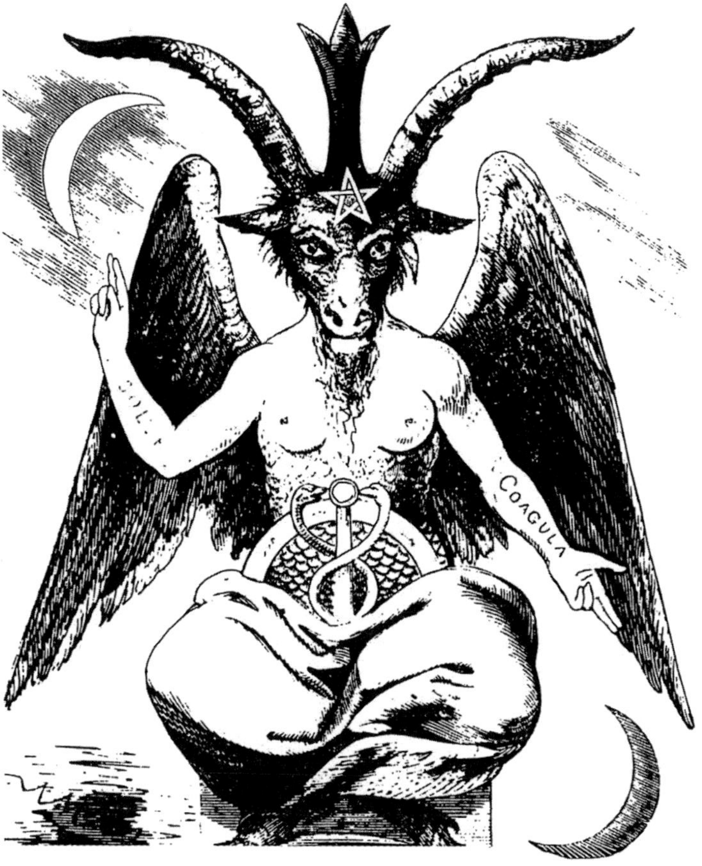

Supreme Court, on June 26, 2013. Once again, the awful "Tammuz 10 anniversary" date holds. America's reprobate mind has won again!

Coming up, the last Tammuz picture: Two men are exchanging wedding rings. Beyond astonishing is that the pattern once more emerges. This is America's complete moral capitulation, defying God's biblical laws (June 26, 2015). Now, so-called "marriage" between a man and a man or a woman and a woman is legalized. A direct affront to God Almighty is now the law of the American land.

Is there a spiritual reason that more Americans died of COVID than in any other country on earth? And why were Americans drastically prohibited from being able to use the very efficacious hydroxy-chloroquine and Ivermectin? These might have saved their lives!

The Return of the Gods gives this interesting summary on page 206: "And so all these landmark events that pushed open the ancient door took place on the exact same date. On top of that, each was the anniversary of the day Stonewall was sealed, which was the beginning of the opening of the door—and which was itself, on the ancient calendar, the day appointed for a man to love a man. And thus, all four events were joined together to the ancient day of the ancient spell." What "spell" does Cahn mean? Is it the spirit of "antichrist" or the "reprobate mind"? God says He will turn willfully sinful men over to a "strong delusion."

We as Christians are supposed to be salt that has not lost its savor, when evil is churning all around us. Habakkuk 2:1–2 says, "I will stand upon my watch, and set me upon the tower, and will watch to see what he will say unto me, and what I shall answer when I am reproved. And the LORD answered me, and said, Write the vision, and make it plain upon tables, that he may run that readeth it." In giving warning, every Christian must tell the truth without compromise.

Americans still have the physical protection of their guns, but serious spiritual erosion has begun. The U.S. has given up allegiance to God's scriptural laws. Churches partnered with Islam, Buddhism, and even pagan witchcraft. In 1973, *Roe v. Wade* gave state-sanctioned approval to murder of more than 60 million unborn, living babes in their mother's wombs. Yet a merciful Almighty God, in A.D. 2022 overturned *Roe v. Wade.* Absolutely no human explanation can account for this political and judicial miracle—only God's patience and mercy, a temporary stay of judgment.

The "Gay Manifesto" of the 1970s, "We Shall Come for Your Sons," is now savagely being fully implemented in an unspeakable way: cutting off the breasts and genitals of young children. This child mutilation is not happening in the Israelite groves. Modern, ***"civilized"*** children's hospitals are doing it! Texas Children's Hospital (the largest U.S. children's hospital) was pioneering in it. Not until a huge storm of publicity arrived in the spring of 2020 did Texas Children's Hospital stop the hellish procedures. [***The biblical cup of evil is now so full, that how can an angry God not act?***]

We return to the question we posed earlier—Are we moving toward (a) coming judgment; or, instead, (b) "end times"? Ancient portals of darkness have now been opened. The most murderous of Satan's demons are bringing with them their vilest practices including "spirit cooking," child trafficking, and cases of child sacrifice. ***As Christians, it is our essential duty to expose such abominations.***

Are we now under God's judgment? Or is it now "end times"? Alan and Pat Franklin's 2006 book, *Goodbye America, Goodbye Britain* (Bible Belt Publishers, page 48), quotes the late evangelist Barry Smith's world government aims he found in an investigation of the secret society Skull and Bones:

» World Dominion "through a New World Order"
» The control of each individual's life from the cradle to the grave.
» A complete change in society.
» No national boundaries.
» The cessation of constitutional protection.
» Complete control of information through the media.

Barry Smith in "Prophecy Club" lectures also called New Zealand "a test case for the New World Order." Alan Franklin in *Goodbye America, Goodbye Britain* (pp. 49–51) also gives us indicators that one-world government may be nearing. Some of these signposts have already come into being. Some of these include:

» Rights will be given by the state and can be suspended by the state. Under the present U.S. Constitution, human rights come from God and are inalienable.
» The state will control or supervise all enterprise through a mass of interlocking laws.
» Lies about so-called global warming will be used to restrict freedom of movement. Public transport will be in, the private car out—this is official policy in Britain, where motoring is incredibly expensive with most of the cost being tax.
» There will be no criticism of the state allowed—a policy already

far advanced in Europe. Freedoms will be curtailed under the guise of "preventing terrorism," a catch-all that gives governments unlimited power.

- There will be no private firearms. America is one of the last places where arms can be borne as a right. This means there will be no chance of fighting back against " Big Brother."
- ... Huge regional governments will control our lives, another trend set by the EU with its unelected regional seats of government. In Britain, the government is trying to line up these regions with the creation of huge new super police forces to cover the same areas.
- Rural areas will become depopulated and there will be fewer private homes outside cities, as the world's population is increasingly funneled into easily-controlled urban areas. Vast areas of countries will be allowed to "go wild" on spurious eco grounds, which has already happened on a large scale in America. Food production will then drop dramatically. Wolves will roam where corn once grew. If this sounds crazy and implausible to you, please check for yourselves: land is being taken out of food production all over America, from Florida, where it is being turned back into swamps as part of the Everglades Restoration Project, to Western states where ranchers are being thrown into jail on accusations that they are grazing cattle on government land without permits. In Britain, open land is almost regarded as sacred and you virtually have more chance of building on the moon than getting a plot to build a family home
- Euthanasia will become legalized, just like abortion.
- The Bible will be banned, as much of it is politically incorrect, and will fall foul of hate crimes legislation.
- There will be no leaving the state and no turning back—not until Jesus returns!

—Elizabeth Cuppett Caverly

CHAPTER TWO

Clandestine Experimentation: Injury and Death to the Populace

The March 14/21, 2022, issue of *Time* magazine showed what was described as a "temporary COVID-19 hospital" in Hong Kong. The rectangular, box-like units resembled shipping containers that had been loaded onto flatbed trucks. Each had bars on what appeared to be its only window. Elizabeth commented that they looked a little like Nazi-era boxcars. I replied, "Yes, but THEY DONT MOVE!" (In other words, this medical/pharma military global police state is now chaining us down in our very homes.)

The great masses cannot conceive that the benevolent government and medical establishment would ever intentionally harm them. Yet, Dutch insurance company Egon reported a 250+ increase in life insurance payouts in the third quarter of 2021, compared to the same period in 2020.

Researcher Karen Kingston on the "Stew Peters Show" on March 2, 2022, gave these highlights:

» We must dump the word "vaccine" when referring to the COVID shots. These are "gene therapies" or "bioweapons," but not true vaccines according to the definition that has always been used in the past.
» The mRNA injection (BNT162b2) can enter human liver cell lines in vitro (Definition of in vitro: "isolated from the living organism and artificially maintained, as in a test tube")—this,

despite claims by the pharmaceutical giants that the "vaccines" remain only at the point of injection.

» A study published in *Current Issues of Molecular Biology* states that "BNT162b2 mRNA is reverse transcribed intracellularly into DNA as fast as in 6 hours." So, the "vaccine" does affect the patient's DNA. This, again, contradicts assurances given by Big Pharma.
» Moderna created this "vaccine" with the HIV virus as one of the components.
» In the Moderna patent, it states, "In another embodiment, the polymer-based self-assembled nanoparticles ... may be fully programmable nanoparticles." What do the developers plan to program in us?
» Karen Kingston found a useful summary of the new research in this field that says that hydrogels (as found in the "vaccines") "are gaining traction with materials from scientists and synthetic biologists who are eyeing the prospect of mass producing these materials via biosynthesis." "Biosynthesis" is using the body (with calcium as the fuel) to make lipid nanoparticles. Fiber networks can be built and signals can be sent to the body. Does this remind us of the fibrous clots that morticians have found in the bodies of the vaccinated?
» The information found in the patents provides an explanation for many of the strange structures seen by scientists under the microscope.
» There are some allegations that intelligent life forms have been injected. These may be given operating instructions remotely. "Spycatcher" was said to be the name for this kind of technology.
» On February 14, 2022, Moderna entered into a fifteen-year contract with Fisher Scientific (Greenville, North Carolina).
» Moderna has opened offices in six countries in Europe and four in Asia. Obviously, Moderna expects to be working on far more than just COVID "vaccines." In the early part of 2023, Dr. Jane Ruby reported that Moderna had fifty new projects (using mRNA) underway.
» The Army, Navy, and CIA conducted joint germ warfare

experiments from 1953 to 1970. Tens of thousands of people in New York City and San Francisco were exposed to airborne germs, some later found to be pathogenic

» In 1969, Henry Kissinger (then national security advisor to President Nixon) directed Defense Secretary Melvin Laird to file a report on the nation's biological weapons capabilities. Laird's deputy director requested $10 million from Congress to "develop and test AIDS-like viruses.[1] [This lends credence that HIV was later intentionally developed.]

» On July 1, 1969, Donald M. MacArthur, director of the U.S. Army Advanced Research Project Agency, testified before a House of Representatives subcommittee. He stated, "Within the next 5 to 10 years, it would probably be possible to make a new infective microorganism which could differ in certain important aspects from any known disease-causing organisms. Most important of these is that it might be refractory [i.e., not yielding to treatment] to the immunological and therapeutic processes."[2]

» By 1975, word had leaked that the Army, in violation of a Geneva accord, was still storing supplies of deadly biological weapons at Fort Detrick in Frederick, Maryland.[3]

» Senator Richard Schweiker, during a hearing of the Senate Subcommittee on Health and Scientific Research, stated, "There have been tests [of biological agents] in my home state of Pennsylvania—in Mechanicsburg, in the Kittatinny and Tuscarora Tunnels of the Pennsylvania Turnpike and along Pennsylvania State Highway 16."[4]

» The U.S. is keeping its stock of smallpox vaccine at Fort Detrick, in spite of the fact that smallpox has been eradicated worldwide since 1980 or before. Officials say the stocks are necessary to permit further research. Such research is banned under various treaties and executive orders.[5]

» Dr. Francis Boyle, author of the Biological Weapons Act, confirmed that "the coronavirus is a biological weapon system which escaped the Wuhan BSL-4 laboratory and broke containment in the local population, spreading uncontrollably."[6]

- Prof. Giuseppe Tritto, president of the World Academy of Biomedical Sciences and Technologies, says that the Wuhan coronavirus (COVID-19) gained cross-species transmission functionality due to genetic engineering that took place at the Wuhan Institute of Virology (WIV), China's only level-four biosafety lab.[7]
- Dr. Anthony Fauci and NIH's role in providing money for "gain of function" research is widely exposed now, as well as the pivotal role of Dr. Ralph Baric at the University of North Carolina. Finally, this summer (2023), Robert F. Kennedy, Jr. bravely revealed to Congress the U.S. government's role in developing bioweapons labs in Ukraine. Magically, right after that, Senator Rand Paul, in August 2023, called for indictment of Fauci. Is this sudden targeting of Fauci at this time at least partially meant to divert the public's attention away from the behemoth CIA–NIH role in establishing the Ukraine bioweapons complex?

In his 2023 book, *Conspiracy 2*, Dr. Dennis Cuddy's chapter, "The Origin of COVID-19, Updated" (p. 179), gives us these crucial facts:

> Dr. Baric and Dr. Zhengli-Li-Shi of the Wuhan Institute of Virology (Lab Level 4), among others, co-authored "A SARS-like cluster of circulating bat coronaviruses shows potential for human emergence," in *Nature Medicine* (November 9, 2015). The article abstract states that "using the SARS-CoV reverse genetics system, we generated and characterized a chimeric virus expressing the spike of bat coronavirus SHCO14 ... and the spike can efficiently use multiple orthology of the SARS receptor human angiotensin converting enzyme 11 (ACE2), replicate efficiently in primary human airway cells. ..." (See also Jef Akst's article in *The Scientist*, November 9, 2015.) Synthetic construction of chimeric mutant and full length SHCO14—CoV was approved by the University of North Carolina Institutional Biosafety Committee and research in this manuscript was supported by grants from the National Science Foundation of China, among others.

Another important article on the subject was "Following the Clues," May 2, 2021, by Nicholas Wade, former *New York Times* science writer. Wade stated, "Dr. Baric had developed and taught Dr. Shi a general method for engineering bat coronaviruses to attack other species. The specific targets were human cells."

Dr. Richard Fleming, in his June 5, 2021, "Event 2021" presentation, discussed a prion-like domain at the receptor binding site. This spike protein in two weeks killed 95 percent of humanized mice. This lethal domain was made by inserting HIV pseudovirus glycoprotein 120 and a Praline Arginine—Arginine Alanine (PRRA)—together.

Dr. Fleming's diagram at his Event 2021 presentation showed the way Dr. Anthony Fauci "passed the 'gain of function' buck on to Peter Daszak. "2005-NIAD Grant RO1A1079231 for $535,156 from September 18, 2008, to June 30, 2013, to Dr. Peter Daszak (Eco Health Alliance CEO) to study factors that explain why some viruses are able to cross the species barrier ... and use a range of in vitro techniques. ..."

In 2016, Dr. Peter Daszak made a statement about a business profits model for big pharma vaccines. "Too often," he stated people ignore an infectious disease until an emergency threshold is reached. "A key driver is the media, and the economics follow the hype. We need to use that hype to our advantage to get to the real issues. Investors will respond if they see profit at the end of the process."

Dr. Dennis Cuddy, the author of *The Power Elite and the Secret Nazi Plan* and *Conspiracy 2* (published by Beacon Street Press) makes a comment that epitomizes what Daszak's statement meant. It really describes the main modus operandi of the New World Order: ***"In other words, use fear to control people."***

Senators like Ron Johnson, Rand Paul, and others for two years have done nothing legislatively to end our government's funding of "gain of function" research. *We have to ask our usual NWO question: **"Why?"***

—Lou Caverly

CHAPTER THREE

Aborted Fetal-Cell COVID Vaccines ... Abomination Begins

"OPERATION WARP SPEED"

A few modern-day journalist watchpersons [Ezekiel 33 and Habakkuk 2:2] were warning of harm very early. In fact, they were raising their concerned voices at the very inception of the COVID pandemic. Note that this NaturalNews.com article was dated June 4, 2020, almost a year before the "Operation Warp Speed" mobile vans were on the road.

> Natural News.com
> June 14, 2020
> by Isabelle Z.
>
> **Some COVID-19 Vaccines Are Being Developed Using Aborted Human Babies' Cell Lines**
>
> A World Health Organization tracker shows that more than 120 vaccine candidates are currently in development, 10 of which have already moved forward to the clinical trial phase ...
>
> Unfortunately, quite a few of the frontrunners are using a human fetal kidney cell line for the development of their trial vaccines. The fetal cell line is known as HEK-293, and it came from the kidney tissue of a baby girl aborted in the Netherlands in 1972. This line is being used in vaccines under development by Moderna, Inovio Pharmaceuticals, Oxford University/AstraZeneca, and CanSino Biologics/Beijing Institute of Technology.

A different human fetal cell line is being used by Janssen, the pharmaceutical division of Johnson and Johnson. The fetal cell line PER.C6 was taken from the retinal tissue of an 18-week-old boy who was aborted in 1985 in the Netherlands.

Much of this vaccine development is being funded by grants from the U.S. government. So far, nearly $2 billion has gone to support the development of vaccines for COVID-19 that use fetal cell lines. A lot of this funding is being awarded through a division of the Department of Health and Human Services called the Biomedical Advanced Research and Development Authority (BARDA).

THE CHURCH HOUSE LARGELY CAPITULATES

Why did God's shepherds not warn people in their churches ahead of time of the moral and physical dangers of taking aborted fetal cell-derived "vaccines" that had only been given hasty emergency-use approval? There was "silence from pastors." Or, they gave out reprobate advice. So, Fox News's medical correspondent Dr. Marc Siegel rose up into a moral advisory role. He soon made quite a Hitlerian pronouncement—to "force-pin" a yellow badge on unvaccinated children!

Not to be outdone, Governor Kathy Hochul stepped out of her statehouse and into the pulpit! At the Christian Cultural Center in Brooklyn, Hochul vaccine-recruited Reverend Bernard and attending worshippers. She said, "God did answer our prayers. He made the smartest men and women, the scientists, the doctors, the researchers, he made men come up with a vaccine, and I wear my 'vaccinated' necklace all the time to say 'I'm vaccinated.' All of you, yes, I know you're vaccinated. You're the smart ones. I need you to be my apostles. I need you to go out and talk about it, and say, 'We owe this to each other.' We love each other. Jesus taught us to love one another, and how do you show that love but to care about each other enough to say please get the vaccine because I love you and I want you to live."

A period of great political and spiritual darkness has begun worldwide, and in America itself. America's Constitution, for now, has been shredded. God's judgment hovers over a largely unrepentant America.

A large number of its pastors advocated for their congregations to take aborted fetal-cell line COVID-19 vaccines. Even more abhorrently, some pastors turned over their sanctuaries to Satan as COVID injection centers.

> Late last year, The Southern Baptist Theological Seminary head Al Mohler urged Southern Baptists to take a Wuhan coronavirus (COVID-19) vaccine because doing so, he suggested, is a way for Christians to "love thy neighbor."
>
> "Pressing against disease and viruses is part of our mandate," Mohler wrote in a lengthy piece that blatantly took the Bible out of context and misappropriated the words of Jesus to push the plandemic agenda. "Medical treatment is an extension of God's common grace and Christians have always understood this."
>
> Pope Francis says coronavirus vaccines made from abortions are "morally acceptable"
>
> The Vatican's official "Congregation for the Doctrine of the Faith," meanwhile, has decided that when "ethically irreproachable COVID-19 vaccines are not available, it is morally acceptable to receive COVID-19 vaccines that have used cell lines from aborted fetuses in their research and production process."
>
> The aborted baby cell line used in J&J's Wuhan flu vaccine is known as PER.C6. It originated in an 18-week-old baby that was murdered back in 1985. These types of fetal cell lines can be used as "miniature 'factories' to generate vast quantities of adenoviruses ... that are used as vehicles to ferry genes from the novel coronavirus that causes COVID-19." According to a June 2020 article published in *Science*.
>
> As it turns out, both the Pfizer-BioNTech and Moderna virus vaccines were made using human fetal cells. In their case, however, these fetal cells were only used during the testing phase of the jabs to determine their "efficacy." [Editor's Note: This is directly contradicted by the earlier June 14 article we quoted that exposed cell line HEK293T from the 1972 aborted Netherlands baby girl.]

> "While neither vaccine company is completely free from any connection to morally compromised cell lines," the bishops added, "in this case, the connection is very remote from the initial evil of the abortion." [*Did the ancient Israelites believe that God would never punish them in those Molech groves—if they stood back one hundred feet, rather than four feet, to toss their babies into the fire?*]
>
> —Ethan Huff, NaturalNews.com

Some Christian doctors of great courage and integrity, including Dr. Stella Emmanuel, Dr. Peter McCullough, and Dr. Jane Ruby have come forward to speak out. Dr. Ruby's latest revelation is shocking, that some vaccine injuries occurred to children too young to have been in the approved age groups. How did this happen during vaccine trials?

Ruby also revealed the Pfizer booster shot is not a smaller dose, but is just the same as its first two doses. Strange to us, also, is the news that these boosters were being heavily pushed on people over fifty who had underlying medical conditions. This CDC recommendation was also applicable to people over sixty-five who had two doses of Pfizer or ones who live in a long-term care facility. Is this Hitler's T-4 euthanasia van rolling again—or what? The old and the handicapped, apparently, are the "useless eaters."

Our suspicions of a global, planned genocide mindset are enhanced by Alice Parks' statement in *Time* magazine, October 11/18, 2021: "Both the World Health Organization and the European Medicines Agency maintain that, so far, the data don't show that boosters are necessary for ***anyone other than people with compromised immune systems."***

Did all Christendom really acquiesce to the COVID shots, and unwittingly endorse the [now-demolished] Georgia Guidestones' depopulation goal to keep the earth's population in balance at ***500 million people***?

Focus on the Family's founder, Dr. James Dobson, to his credit, did take a moderate stand against using aborted fetal cell-derived vaccines. Roman Catholic archbishop Carlo Maria Vigano admirably spoke out consistently against this pragmatic new vaccine adaptation of evil.

How did other key Protestant and Roman Catholic clerical leaders react to this moral question? Dr. Franklin Graham advised his flock to indeed be like Jesus and take the shots. Sadly, he himself became one of the post-COVID shot victims who developed myocarditis, a grave heart inflammation. CBN's Gordon Roberson advised getting the shots. Russell Moore, president of the Ethics and Religious Liberty Commission of the Southern Baptist Convention (SBC), stated, "We should oppose authorizing or funding research rooted in the taking of innocent human life. That does not mean, though, that people must shun medical treatments that can save lives because they were discovered through ***means*** which ***we would not necessarily approve."***

[Doesn't the Bible say a little bit of leaven leavens the whole lump? This kind of "moral pragmatism" reminds us of news a few years ago that a U.K. hospital was burning aborted fetuses for fuel. No doubt the "depopulation" globalists would call this hospital move "pragmatic" and cost-cutting.]

BRAVE CHRISTIAN—MELISSA STRICKLER
PFIZER WHISTLEBLOWER
"We Want to Avoid Having the Information on the Fetal Cells Floating Out There"

[New York – Oct. 6, 2021] Project Veritas released the fifth video in its COVID vaccine investigation series today featuring a sit-down interview with Pfizer insider, Melissa Strickler. She leaked internal emails that show corporate executives telling staff to be secretive about the use of human fetal tissue in laboratory testing of the COVID vaccine. Pfizer's Chief Scientific Officer, Philip Dormitzer, admits aborted fetus tissue is used in the company's vaccine program, but that employees should just stick with Pfizer's polished narrative omitting any mention of aborted fetal tissue to avoid any issues with the public.

» Vanessa Gelman, Pfizer Senior Director of Worldwide Research: "From the perspective of corporate affairs, we want to avoid having the information on fetal cells floating out there. ... The risk of communicating this right now outweighs any potential benefit we could see, particularly with general members of the public who may take this information and use it in ways we may not want out there. We have not received any questions from policy makers or media on this issue in the last few weeks, so we want to avoid raising this if possible."

» Gelman: "We have been trying as much as possible to not mention the fetal cell lines. ... One or more cell lines with an origin that can be traced back to human fetal tissue has been used in laboratory tests associated with the vaccine program."

» Philip Dormitzer, Pfizer Chief Scientific Officer: "HEK293T cells, used for the IVE assay, are ultimately derived from an aborted fetus," Dormitzer said. "On the other hand, the Vatican doctrinal committee has confirmed that they consider it acceptable for Pro-Life believers to be immunized. Pfizer's official statement couches the answer well and is what should be provided in response to an outside inquiry."

» Melissa Strickler, Pfizer Insider and Manufacturing quality Auditor: "They're being so deceptive in their emails, its almost like it is in the final vaccine, it just made me not trust it."

» Strickler: I came to Project Veritas because "I have no one else to turn to when my own company won't be honest with me. What I was told to do was to trust Project Veritas and to go with you guys by lawmakers, by lawyers."

— www.projectveritas.com, October 6, 2021

[More from Melissa: mRNA Acting as CRISPR DNA; Luciferase]

October 15, 2021, *LifeSite*'s Jim Hale interviewed courageous "about-to-be-terminated" Pfizer employee Melissa Strickler. Strickler, a Christian, was morally compelled, she said, to come forward, revealing shocking Pfizer "insider" e-mails to Project Veritas.

Victoria Gelman, Pfizer senior director of worldwide research, was caught on an e-mail advising the need to cover up the fetal-cell derivation issue of the Pfizer COVID vaccine. Pfizer chief scientific officer Phillip Dormancer's e-mail also came under scrutiny. Revealed were Pfizer research details using HEK-293T cells. Strickler explained, "These are human embryonic kidney cells from an aborted fetus from the 1970s. These cells never stop replicating, unlike the way normal cells die. They use these 'cancerous cells' to see how the vaccine they're working on affects our human cells."

Strickler emphasized that mRNA technology is never mentioned to be, in actuality, "CRISPR technology" that "edits your DNA." She also suspects strongly that Bill Gates' "Luciferase" (SM102) is a component of the Pfizer vaccine. The fact the vaccine "glows," she says, could come from only two causes: graphene oxide and "Luciferase." The latter has some components akin to the makeup of lightning bugs' light flashes. Pfizer admitted "Luciferase" was used in the experimental trials, but Strickler believes it was in the final version as well, because, after all, the "final" vaccine is still "experimental." This Luciferase "glow," Strickler explains, will identify someone as being vaccinated.

—Divided Kingdom Radio Monologue, October 19, 2021

Strickler embodies the courage and sacrifice of a true Christian. Though losing her job, she stood heroically, witnessing for Christ against great evil powers. Melissa said she was compelled by God to come forward to tell the truth she knew. She believes we may very well be living in the time of the Revelation 18 warning: "The whole world was deceived by 'spells.'" Melissa explained that this word, "spells" in Greek, is "*pharmakeia*"!

—*Elizabeth Cuppett Caverly*

CHAPTER FOUR

"Country Roads" ... T-4 Comes to Appalachia

CHARLESTON BIBLE CENTER CHURCH INJECTION SITE AND MIKAELA'S STORY

Lou: Seventy-seven years ago, top American military brass, including Generals Eisenhower and Patton, walked into the literal hell on earth of places like Dachau. One or more of them vomited at the unimaginable horror of human corpses stacked high like firewood. The feeble skeletons of humanity, still barely alive, hollow-eyed, staring at them, were beyond imagination—proof of the Nazis' murderous insanity. Crosses in most German churches had long since been replaced by swastikas. In our day, Pope Francis had a one-on-one high-level meeting with Pfizer's CEO.

There is something really evil, it seems, that was let loose by Satan, in 2021, in that beautiful state that John Denver celebrated in the song with the words, "Country roads take me home." Home in that West Virginia fall foliage paradise is now Hades.

Elizabeth: Yes, Lou. *Time* magazine for July5/July 12, 2021, has an article entitled "The Home Stretch." Situated in Kanawah County, West Virginia, this was the final lap for coercion. Church members were commanded by visiting "special pastor," and so-called Christian, Dr. Francis Collins (former NIH head): "Roll up your sleeves!" Get all those poor Appalachian adults and children injected. Kanawah health officials were even making house calls ... "Country roads, take me home." ...

The article opens with these words: "'Hi sweetie,' Dr. Sherri Young says to the 13-year-old rolling up her sleeve and giggling nervously, who also happens to be her daughter. 'Are you ready?' Young uncaps a syringe and pokes it into her daughter's waiting arm. It's May 14, only a few days after the U.S. Food and Drug Administration greenlighted the Pfizer Bio-N-Tech vaccine for 12–15-year-olds, and Young is trying to set an example."

Lou: We are informed that this health officer called for families to come to other West Virginia community health clinics like this one that was a drive-through set up in a church parking lot a few miles outside downtown Charleston.

Elizabeth: Dr. Young is shown getting ready to inoculate her Kanawah County Sheriff's security guard, Doug Beasley, assigned to her, "after threats on health offices around the country during the pandemic."

Lou: No Hitlerian T-4 euthanasia van is required to pick up the handicapped victim/targets in this impoverished Appalachian county. Well-meaning parents often can be tragically misled. The *Time* article states *"Allison Bungard helps her son, Andrew, 13, who has cerebral palsy and Factor V Leiden thrombophilia, receive his shot at a vaccine clinic in Charleston."*

Then, too, there is the convenience of getting the jab right where you live. In fact, *Time* magazine next shows an octogenarian, "Dana Campbell, playing the harmonica before ***being vaccinated in his home*** in Elkview."

Elizabeth: I wonder whether Dana Campbell is still on Earth six months later; or is he a post-clot shot statistic? One like those in many obituaries I read in Maryland newspapers. White and black men and women in their twenties to seventies who passed away either "peacefully" or "unexpectedly" at home. A scary picture accompanied *Time*'s statement: *"Cheridan Quigley of Saint Albans is vaccinated at Charleston's Bible Center Church on June 4."*

Lou: Notice a close-up of Ms. Quigley's face. Her look of utter horror. She was wearing big glasses. Something about the magazine lighting and her one raised eyebrow seemed to distort her right eye so that it looked a lot like the veritable *"All-Seeing Eye of Horus." Remember, this Molech inoculation was done at God's sacred house! Charleston Bible Center Church.* Not the swastika here; no, the caduceus—the two serpents interwoven around the staff.

Elizabeth: Lou, the Nazi Joseph Mengele-days are back again, too, right here right in Huntington, West Virginia's Mercy Hospital.

Lou: That's right. On January 20, 2022, "The Stew Peters Show" interviewed heroic West Virginia mother Mikaela Hughes. The program first gave an update on the case of Scott Quinar, who had been held hostage and refused efficacious COVID treatments by Minnesota's Mercy Hospital. Legal tactics won so that Scott had now been airlifted to Texas, where the withheld treatments would now be administered. Stew Peters stated that this sort of quiet euthanasia was going on in thousands of paid-off hospitals that get $40,000 per patient put on a ventilator and $100,000 for each ventilator death!

Mother Mikaela Hughes told that her 32-year-old son, Charles, a very fit father of four and a paramedic, traveled to St. Mary's Hospital in Huntington, West Virginia, just to get an inhaler for his asthma. But once inside the door, the hospital made him get two COVID tests, both negative. They wouldn't let him go home. (We wonder whether this was using bodily restraints, not just words of intimidation.) For, his mother recounts, Charles had a panic attack—possibly just an asthma attack from the stress. So, they put him in the ICU and, despite his protests, put him on a ventilator and gave him Remdesivir.

Courageous Mikaela fought hard for her son. St. Mary's told her he would only be on the ventilator for two days. But more than fifty-two days passed! Charles began to decline, with the drugs given to him being suspected of causing a heart attack. The mother was kept away from visiting her son.

A patient advocate let it slip that Charles had been double vaccinated for COVID while there. The mother cried, "But he was exempt on religious grounds by choice!"

The talk-show host commented that if this was done against his will, it is a criminal act. (When the mother demanded to know when these vaccinations occurred, the patient advocate just hemmed and hawed.) Charles tried to pull out the ventilator and doctors increased paralytic or paralyzing drugs. He mouthed the words to his mother, "Out! out!" After all of this horror, the original test Charles had requested, the test for bacterial pneumonia, was given. It came back positive.

Elizabeth: The mother, Mikaela, thinks the covert vaccinations were done to her son while he was on the ventilator. Of course, while he was given Remdesivir, Charles was denied Ivermectin. The doctor in charge kept telling the hapless mother, "Your son is dying." Dr. Segamarsi (spelling?) was the doctor treating Charles. One morning he allegedly told Charles, "You won't be going home for two to three years. You'll be in a nursing home."

But by that evening—as publicity grew—Dr. Segamarsi had released Charles to the care of a Dr. Cohn. Stew Peters commented, "This is savage—if they vaccinated him against his will." Another physician who had personally escaped from a communist country said, "This is just like Nazi Germany!" Mikaela remarked, "I think they were trying to kill him. This is sad. People are just commodities. It's going on all over the world."

Lou: Protect your families. Do not go to the hospital unless you must. As Ezekiel 33 commands, Elizabeth and I must warn you of these horrific things that must be stopped. We must pray, repent and beseech God to stop this killing!

— Lou and Elizabeth Caverly
Radio Dialogue
Late January 2022

CHAPTER FIVE

The Children's Horrors Begin

The first article we quote appeared at the early onset of "Operation Warp Speed."

DISNEYLAND CONVERTED INTO MASS COVID-19 VACCINATION SITE

(Ethan Huff, *Natural News,* Thursday, January 14, 2021)

The Disneyland Resort in Anaheim, Calif., which has been closed to the public for nearly a year due to the COVID-19 crisis, has been converted into a so-called "Super POD site" for the mass administration of vaccines.

In partnership with President Donald Trump's "Operation Warp Speed" program, Disneyland was transformed into "the first Super Point-of-Dispensing (POD) site for COVID-19 vaccines in Orange County," officials indicated.

One of five that has been set up throughout the area, the Disneyland Super POD site is being furnished with enough injections to jab thousands of people daily, until eventually millions have received Big Pharma's untested messenger RNA (mRNA) technology inside their bodies.

"The Disneyland Resort, the largest employer in the heart of Orange County, has stepped up to host the county's first Super POD site—undertaking a monumental task in our vaccination distribution process," said acting Chairman Andrew Do, from the First District, in a statement about the new program. Doug Chaffee, Orange County's

Supervisor, added that these Super POD sites are "absolutely critical in stopping this deadly virus."

Just seven months later, the "Sanger to Hitler move" is made. The Aussie tots won't have any cute kiddie rides to camouflage depopulation medical equipment. (Another later chapter in this book mentions that the U.S. DoD played an initial role in setting up Australia's COVID quarantine gulag.)

AUSTRALIA LAUNCHES STADIUM-SCALE COVID DEATH SHOT PROCESSING CENTER TO INJECT 24,000 CHILDREN WITHOUT PARENTAL CONSENT

(Ethan Huff, *Natural News,* August 20, 2021)

Brad Hazzard [What? *His name is a coincidental synonym for "harm"!*], the Minister for Health and Medical Research in New South Wales, Australia, has announced that 24,000 children will be "vaccinated" for the Wuhan coronavirus (COVID-19) ***without their parents' permission*** [emphasis added] at the Qudos Bank Arena in Sydney.

In order to attend school in the upcoming term, students in Australia are having to get injected for the Chinese virus. To make it as easy as possible for them to roll up their sleeves, the government rented out an entire sports stadium for quick in-and-out jabbing.

"Maybe mum and dad can drop you," Hazzard stated during a press conference. "This is a *'golden opportunity'* for Australia's youth to get the shots, including those *WHO DO NOT WANT THEIR PARENTS KNOWING ABOUT IT. MAKE SURE THEY STAY OUTSIDE THE ARENA because we don't want too many people OBVIOUSLY MILLING AROUND inside the arena. Make some arrangements for [someone] to wait outside for you.*" Hazzard added that *no parents or adults of any kind will be allowed inside the Qudos Bank Arena or anywhere in Sydney Olympic Park while their children are getting injected.*

"I want to stress that to the mums and dads, your children will be well looked after inside. When they arrive, they'll be LITERALLY USHERED.

We'll have nurses, we'll have some of the youth command, we'll have some of the YOUNG POLICE from various operations with the police there just to guide them through as to where they go. ***They'll be looked after every moment*** *inside the stadium and they'll be well cared for so mums and dads feel* ***secure."***

Australia's Department of Defence (DOD) put up a tweet [https://twitter.com/DefenceAust/status/1427465254502555648] depicting *SOLDIERS escorting children around the arena and in and out of white tents for their PFIZER INJECTION treatments.* Some of the soldiers were seen dispensing what appeared to be hand sanitizer into children's hands while directing them as to where they should go. Once inside the arena, children were greeted with a large screen showing Australian Liberal Party leader Gladys Berejiklian spewing propaganda about how getting injected will keep everyone ***"safe"*** against the Chinese flu while helping to ***"flatten the curve."*** [This article also quoted Australia's Department of Defense website, August 17, 2021, stating the bank center could process up to 30,000 vaccines a week.]

The Australian government continues to tell the population *there that getting injected is the "ticket to freedom"* [https://www.naturalnews.com/2021-05-26-yes-COVID-vaccines-are-spreading-variants.html], suggesting that *the only thing the "UNVACCINATED" have to look forward to is SECOND-CLASS TREATMENT AND SLAVERY.* [Editor's note: The article stated at least **two students who were ushered into the Sydney arena died after receiving their injections.**]

"This Brett Hazzard is the modern-day Mengele; he will be receiving a major reckoning. God said: 'If anyone causes one of these little ones—those who believe in me—to stumble, it would be better for them to have a large millstone hung around their neck and to be drowned in the depths of the sea.'"

CHILDREN'S HORROR HOUR CALENDAR

January 2021, Disneyland Resort, Anaheim; August, 2021, Qudos Bank Arena, Sydney, Australia; July, 2023, NEW SATANIC SACRIFICE TO MOLECH CARTOON

HELLISH HEADLINE, SUMMER, 2023

Disney-Produced Cartoon Features Illuminati-Style Robed Elites Drinking Blood, Sacrificing People and Worshipping an All-Seeing Eye

(Steve Watson, Infowars.com, July 12, 2023)

A new Disney cartoon series is based around a cult of robed elites drinking blood, carrying out rituals including human sacrifice and worshipping an all-seeing eye symbol.

[The "Death Gestalt" of this chapter came full circle with some horrifying statistics. National File's Frankie Stockes, writing on July 2, 2022, documented a 500 percent increase in orders for child-size coffins—just in the last seven months!]

A casket salesman blew the whistle on the massive spike in post-COVID jab child mortality on the Stew Peters Show. Casket salesman Mick Haddock described the massive spike in orders for child-size caskets experienced by his family's manufacturing business. The post-COVID vaccine spike, he says, is the first time in his family's 30-plus years of business that they've sold children's coffins in bulk. "My family business is casket manufacturing in North America. We received 2 bulk orders for sub-5-foot units (children size) in less than 6 months," Haddock tweeted in response to the initial post. "Never in 30+ years of business have we ever sold child-size coffins in bulk."

His family's business deals with major distribution companies all over the US and Canada, including Costco. The products are then sold to retailers and to funeral homes all over North America. "The smaller size orders have never been so popular," Haddock told Stew Peters of the massive spike in children's orders, adding that sales of adult caskets have spiked big time since 2020 as well. "I would like to mention that all casket sales are up dramatically in the last two years. Call it what you will, ***magic*** or the ***vaccine***, but something has happened that is causing an unprecedented amount of deaths," Haddock went on to say [emphasis added]. "What we're seeing here are intended consequences," Peters concluded of the massive post-vaccine death wave.

Putting into perspective just how massive an uptick in children's coffin orders his family business has experienced, Haddock told Peters that the orders have risen upwards of 500% in the past seven months. "We went through an average of say, 50, 60 [child-size caskets] a year. The last order was 200 and the next order after that was 250. We've now basically sold 5 years' worth of stock in 7 months."

MORE CHILDREN'S HORRORS

3-Year-Old Girl Dies of Heart Attack One Day After Taking COVID Vaccine

Another girl dies of heart attack caused by the vaccine that has now been made into a mandate even upon children who are under zero threat of getting severe reactions from the virus. The girl's parents are quite devastated and have taken to the media to express their grief.

According to her mother, a three-year-old girl in Argentina died of a heart attack the day after taking the COVID vaccine that was mandatory for her just to start kindergarten.

Miryam Suárez told Telefe Tucumán that the vaccine and legislative compulsion killed her child, Ámbar, who had previously been healthy and "full of life. I pre-enrolled her in school so that next year she would enter kindergarten, because now they force you when it comes to the vaccine," Suárez said. "She was healthy. She was fine. She was not ill and didn't have COVID."

On December 16, Suárez accompanied her daughter to go and get immunized. After slumping whilst playing with her friends, Ámbar died the very next day. "She just collapsed and fell." Suárez exclaimed, "I cannot believe it."

The authorities "demand so much that they get the vaccine, and I know that the vaccine killed my three-year-old daughter," the distraught mother explained. "She was fine. She did not have any health issues, nor was she a sick child. She was healthy, full of life.

This government that forces you [to get the vaccine] killed my three-year-old baby."

— Great Game India, January 6, 2022

Dec. 14, 2020 to Nov. 26, 2021: 5-Year-Old Died 4 Days After Pfizer Shot, CDC VAERS Data Show

U.S. VAERS data from Dec. 14, 2020, to Nov. 26, 2021 for 5- to 11-year-olds show:

» 2,586 adverse events, including 34 rated as serious and 2 reported deaths. One death occurred in an 11-year-old girl from Georgia vaccinated Sept. 14, prior to the authorization of Pfizer's COVID vaccine in the 5 to 11 age group.
» The second death (VAERS I.D. 1890705) occurred in a 5-year-old girl who died four days after receiving her first dose of Pfizer.
» 1,581 adverse events have been reported in the 5 to 11 age group since Nov. 1.

U.S. VAERS data from Dec. 14, 2020, to Nov. 26, 2021 for 12 – to 17-year-olds show:

» 23,871 adverse events, including 1,453 rated as serious and 31 reported deaths.
» The most recent death involves a 16-year-old girl from Georgia (VAERS I.D. 1865389) who died reportedly from a heart condition and multi-organ failure two days after receiving Pfizer's COVID vaccine.
» 60 reports of anaphylaxis among 12- to 17-year-olds where the reaction was life-threatening, required treatment or resulted in death—with 96% of cases attributed to Pfizer's vaccine.
» 563 reports of myocarditis and pericarditis (heart inflammation) with 553 cases attributed to Pfizer's vaccine.
» 139 reports of blood clotting disorders, with all cases attributed to Pfizer.

—Megan Redshaw, Children's Health Defense

Jill Biden Sings Happy Birthday to Masked 3-Year-Old on His Way to Get Jabbed at Vaccine Clinic

(Alicia Powe, The Gateway Pundit, July 11, 2022)

Jill Biden celebrated a masked three-year-old boy's COVID-19 vaccination on his birthday during her visit to a vaccine clinic to promote the jab for children.

Following her visit at the Henrico Health Department East Clinic in Virginia, she shared a video of the moment on social media to promote coronavirus vaccines for children. *"I am so glad Dr. Ashish Jha* (COVID-19 Response Team Coordinator) *and I could celebrate your* ***COVID-19 vaccine*** *— and your* ***3rd birthday!***" [*Afterthought?*]

On the website picture, the First Lady is leaning toward the tiny blond 3-year-old boy. She has her arms and fingers widely outstretched, as though to clutch him closer. The boy looks frozen—*scared*, with his arms tightly at his sides. *MAYBE THIS CHILD INSTINCTIVELY KNOWS HE DOESN'T WANT TO BE REELED IN.* [*Pharmakeia* witchcraft?]

As Biden greeted staff and parents of children under 5 who awaited vaccination she assured, *"The relief is finally here—a vaccine for our* ***youngest*** *children. Thank you for coming in today," she said. "Thank you for doing this and protecting your children."* She praised parents for masking their children. *"You* ***wrestled*** *tiny little masks on your children who couldn't understand them.* [STRONG-ARMED TINY TOTS?] *I know that it's been hard, but you've done an amazing job."*

She also thanked the media for helping to spread the message and encouraging parents to vaccinate their young children. ***"We couldn't do this without you—we couldn't get the word out,"*** she said.

—*Elizabeth Cuppett Caverly*

CHAPTER SIX

Spike Protein Causing Phenomenon:"Died Suddenly"?

In 2021 Divided Kingdom Radio reported this important headline—"Salk Institute Says Spike Protein Causes Blood Clots, Strokes, Heart Attacks." Mike Adams wrote an excellent article about *The Circulation Research* science paper's findings:

> The prestigious Salk Institute published a bombshell scientific article revealing that the SARS-CoV-2 spike protein is what's actually causing vascular damage in COVID patients and COVID vaccine recipients, promoting the strokes, heart attacks, migraines, blood clots and other harmful reactions that have already killed thousands of Americans. (source: VAERS.hhs.gov) Critically, all four COVID vaccine brands currently in widespread use either inject patients with the spike protein or, via mRNA technology, instruct the patient's own body to manufacture spike proteins and release them into their own blood. This floods the patient's body with the very spike protein that the Salk Institute has now identified as the smoking gun cause of vascular damage and related events (such as blood clots, which are killing many people who take the vaccines).
>
> Put simply, it means the vaccines were designed to contain the very element that's killing people.
>
> The false assumption of the vaccine industry and its propagandists is that the spike protein is "inert" and harmless. The Salk Institute proves this assumption to be dangerously inaccurate.
>
> —Mike Adams, Natural News .com, May 7, 2021

Now, more about the findings in the article. Mike Adams described details that the Salk Institute published:

In an article entitled, "The Novel Coronavirus' Spike Protein Plays Additional Key Role in Illness," published on April 30, 2021, the Salk Institute warns that, "Salk researchers and collaborators show how the protein damages cells, confirming COVID-19 as a primarily vascular disease."

The Salk Institute article refers to a science paper published in *Circulation Research:* "SARS-CoV-2 Spike Protein Impairs Endothelial Function via Downregulation of ACE 2."

This paper is the first to document how spike proteins—even ones lacking an active virus—cause vascular destruction by binding to ACE2 receptors and harming of the cellular mitochondria. An excerpt from the vital paper explains:

> *We learn that "the researchers created a 'pseudovirus' that was surrounded by SARS-CoV-2 classic crown of spike proteins, but did not contain any actual virus. Exposure to this pseudovirus resulted in damage to the lungs and arteries of an animal model—proving that the spike protein alone was enough to cause disease. Tissue samples showed inflammation in endothelial cells lining the pulmonary artery walls.*
>
> *"The team then replicated this process in the lab, exposing healthy endothelial cells (which line arteries) to the spike protein. They showed that the spike protein damaged the cells by binding ACE2. This binding disrupted ACE2's molecular signaling to mitochondria (organelles that generate energy for cells), causing the mitochondria to become damaged and fragmented."*
>
> *SARS-CoV-1 [Spike] protein promotes lung injury by decreasing the level of ACE2 in the infected lungs. In the current study, we show that S protein alone can damage vascular endothelial cells (ECs) by downregulating ACE2 and consequently inhibiting mitochondrial function.*
>
> *We next studied the impact of S protein on mitochondrial function. Confocal images of ECs treated with S1 protein revealed increased mitochondrial fragmentation, indicating altered mitochondrial dynamics ...*

Moreover, ACE2-L overexpression caused increased basal acidification rate, glucose-induced glycolysis, maximal glycolytic capacity, and glycolytic reserve (Figure [D], ii). Also, ECs incubated with S1 protein had attenuated mitochondrial function but increased glycolysis, when compared with control cells treated with IgG ...

... our data reveals that S protein alone can damage endothelium, manifested by impaired mitochondrial function and eNOS activity but increased glycolysis. It appears that S protein in ECs increases redox stress which may lead to AMPK deactivation, MDM2 upregulation, and ultimately ACE2 destabilization.

Mike Adams' May 7 article continues:

> The Circulation Research article does not mention that COVID-19 vaccines are injecting patients with the very same spike protein that was studied, but this fact is widely known and even touted by the vaccine industry. The upshot of this research is that COVID vaccines are inducing vascular disease and directly causing injuries and deaths stemming from blood clots and other vascular reactions. This is all caused by the spike protein that's deliberately engineered into the vaccines.
>
> mRNA vaccines transform the human body's own cells into spike protein factories, spilling deadly spike protein particles into the bloodstream.
>
> A growing number of researchers are also finding that these spike proteins appear to be "shedding" or transmitting from the vaccinated to the unvaccinated, causing adverse reactions in people who were never vaccinated themselves, but who have spent time close to other people who were.
>
> The technology behind this is called "self-replicating vaccines," and it was pioneered by doctors and scientists working under the racist Apartheid regime of South Africa. There, medical researchers designed race-specific, weaponized, self-replicating vaccines that were designed to spread through the Black population of South Africa and

exterminate the masses who posed a threat to the ruling technocratic elite.

Today, we are all the targets of these weapon systems as globalists seek to exterminate human populations on a global scale, regardless of skin color or country of origin.

Just this year, the Johns Hopkins Bloomberg School of Public Health has celebrated this self-replicating vaccine technology and is calling for it to be used to achieve global mass vaccination, augmented by surveillance drones and AI robots that enforce vaccine compliance (probably at gunpoint).

In effect, mRNA vaccines function as bioweapons factories that turn human beings into biological weapon manufacturing and transmission hubs, spreading vascular damage and death to the entire population, including those who were not yet vaccinated. All COVID vaccines are risky medical experiments, yet the oblivious masses are brainwashed and told the vaccines have all been "approved" as safe and effective

The FDA has not granted therapeutic approval for any COVID-19 vaccine, and no long-term trials have been completed to show COVID-19 vaccines as safe and effective. Rather, the FDA granted experimental authorization use in the USA, which admits that those who take the vaccines are participating in a risky medical experiment with unknown consequences.

Those who take the vaccine are often brainwashed or deceived by the lying corporate media which falsely claims COVID vaccines have been "approved" by the FDA and have harmed no one. The government's own VAERS data at VAERS.hhs.gov proves otherwise.

The medical science establishment that pushes vaccines is now engaged in Holocaust-level crimes against humanity. Josef Mengele would be proud. (He was eventually executed by public hanging for his crimes against humanity.)

THE DR. DREW SPIKE PROTEIN INTERVIEW

In December 2022, Dr. Drew of "Ask Dr. Drew" interviewed pathologist and virologist Dr. Ryan Cole. Cole said that in his opinion the spike proteins can travel anywhere in the body after the vaccine is administered. That includes, he remarked, in the brain. Dr. Drew asked, "Is it in the brain matter? Is it the white matter? Where in the brain?"

"Wherever the lipid nanoparticle distributes—and it does get through the blood-brain barrier and we know S1, the spike protein, gets through as well."

Next, Cole showed Dr. Drew's audience slides demonstrating spike protein effects as they interacted with lymphocytes. "That spike protein causes the lymphocytes to chew a hole in the aorta," Cole said. "This is the biggest blood vessel coming off your heart. When that ruptures, you're gone in minutes. So that's another example of what deposited spike protein and the induced inflammation can do." Cole believes that a very concerning fact is that spike proteins are very persistent. It takes the body almost forever to rid itself of them, if that is even possible.

THE INHIBITION OF DNA DAMAGE REPAIR

The following article is from information contained in the journal *Viruses* entitled "Crucial Info on Spike Protein Effects."

(Ethan Huff, NaturalNews.com, November 5, 2021)

> A study published in the open-access journal *Viruses* looked at the effects of SARS-CoV-2 spike proteins—these are found in (Johnson & Johnson, AstraZeneca) or created by (Pfizer-BioNTech, Moderna) Fauci Flu shots—on the human body. What was discovered might send shivers down your spine. In essence, injection spike proteins inhibit natural DNA damage repair, which is an essential component of the body's adaptive immune response. Jab spike proteins localize themselves in the nucleus of cells and block key DNA repair proteins such as BRCA1 and 53BP1 from doing their job.
>
> "Our findings reveal a potential molecular mechanism by which the spike protein might impede adaptive immunity and underscore the potential side effects of full-length spike-based vaccines." Once injected into the body, the study further explains, spike proteins "hijack

and dysregulate the host cellular machinery to replicate, assemble, and spread progeny viruses."

In a worst-case scenario, the result is a drastic decline in T cells, helper T cells and suppressor T cells, all of which are needed to fight off malignant cells that, if left unchecked, can cause tumors to develop. "As two critical host surveillance systems, the immune and DNA repair systems are the primary systems that higher organisms rely on for defense against diverse threats and tissue homeostasis," the study reads.

"Emerging evidence indicates that these two systems are interdependent, especially during lymphocyte development and maturation." As certain key functions of DNA repair degrade due to said spike proteins, both T and B cells take a huge hit, leading to immunodeficiency. This means that injecting spike proteins into the body *damages* the immune system.

"If DNA damage cannot be properly repaired, it will contribute to the amplification of viral infection-induced pathology," the study further warns. The fact that COVID "vaccine" spike proteins accumulate in cell nuclei is particularly problematic because this is where the most critical aspects of DNA repair take place. In order to ensure genome stability, all of the necessary components for DNA repair and maintenance must converge in the nuclei as designed. This cannot happen, however, when spike proteins get in the way [https://www.naturalnews.com/2021-11-02-COVID-vaccines-inhibit-dna-repair-cause-cancer.html].

"NHEJ repair and homologous recombination (HR) repair are two major DNA repair pathways that not only continuously monitor and ensure genome integrity but are also vital for adaptive immune cell functions," the study explains about one such DNA repair component that is negatively impacted by the presence of spike proteins.

It was observed that spike proteins cause certain DNA repair proteins to either over- or under-express themselves, which in turn diminishes the efficiency of NHEJ and other DNA repair components from activating as they should.

[Editor's Note: Another fact of grave concern is the finding that the full-length type of spike protein causes the most damage, and that it is the very type used in both adenovirus and mRNA injections. This diabolical "seeding" of possible gradual deaths, "not all at once," will help the public to be unaware. This "Died Suddenly" time bomb may continue through 2025 and even beyond ...]

—*Elizabeth Cuppett Caverly*

CHAPTER SEVEN

Early Warning of Artificial Intelligence— The Coming of the A.I. "Tin Man"

Excerpts from: "Vaccines: an ideal covert op to genetically reengineer humans"

(Jon Rappoport, PrisonPlanet.com, July 13, 2015)

I want to extend the remarks I made about vaccines the other day.

The reference is the *New York Times*, 3/15/15, *"Protection Without a Vaccine."* It describes the frontier of research. Here are key quotes that illustrate the use of synthetic genes to "protect against disease," while changing the genetic makeup of humans. This is not science fiction.

"By delivering synthetic genes into the muscles of the [experimental] monkeys, the scientists are essentially re-engineering the animals to resist disease."

"'The sky's the limit,' said Michael Farzan, an immunologist at Scripps and lead author of the new study."

"The first human trial based on this strategy—called immunoprophylaxis by gene transfer, or I.G.T.—is underway, and several new ones are planned."

"I.G.T. is altogether different from traditional vaccination. It is instead a form of gene therapy. Scientists isolate the genes that produce powerful antibodies against certain diseases and then synthesize artificial versions. The genes are placed into viruses and injected into human tissue, usually muscle."

Here is the punchline: "The viruses invade human cells with their DNA payloads, and the synthetic gene is incorporated into the recipient's own DNA. If all goes well, the new genes instruct the cells to begin manufacturing powerful antibodies."

Read that again: "the synthetic gene is incorporated into the recipient's own DNA." Alteration of the human genetic makeup. Not just a "visit." "Permanent residence."

The *Times* article taps Dr. David Baltimore for an opinion:

"Still, Dr. Baltimore says that he envisions that some people might be leery of a vaccination strategy that means altering their own DNA, even if it prevents a potentially fatal disease."

Yes, some people might be leery. If they have two or three working brain cells ...

With vaccines that permanently alter human genetic makeup on the horizon, and given the corporate and government-agency penchant for secrecy, we are already inhabiting the Brave New World. It's not a distant prospect.

Every genetic innovation is aimed at *bringing us closer to a stimulus-response world,* and further away from freedom.

Which is why the defense of freedom becomes ever more vital.

CHAPTER EIGHT

Part One: God's Created Human Turned into A.I. Operating System

[We have met Pogo. And he is us. The U.S. government!] Not the Chi-Coms alone; or simply Pope Francis and the Vatican; Bill Gates and his foundation; Klaus Schwab and the WEF; or even the formidable EU. (After all, Archbishop Carlo Maria Vigano reports the EU has these graphene oxide projects planned.)

No, Dr. Ariyana Love (Brighteon.com, Monday, December 6, 2021), adds the missing all-American puzzle piece. Who could have thought that DARPA (Defense Advanced Research Projects Agency) developed the hydrogels patented by Moderna in patent #8415325B2? Pfizer, Johnson and Johnson, and BioNTech, according to Dr. Love, use these hydrogels.

Love presents some stunning research findings: at least seven groups, including the U. of Almeria, used methods such as optical and electron microscopy, as well as dark field spectroscopy and chemical analysis to determine the presence of graphene oxide and graphene hydroxide in the vaccines, as well as authenticating a wireless nanotech sensor. Hydrogels are made from graphene oxide. Quantum data are also referred to in the Moderna patent. These are all made from graphene oxide. According to Dr. Andrew Nowak, commenting on the graphene oxide, *"This is like razor blades cutting people up!"*

In addition, she reveals, 100 percent of the patents mention gene editing. All but one of them refers to gene editing using synthetic DNA (also called complementary DNA). The U.S. Supreme Court ruled in 2013 that CDNA can be patented. (God-given human DNA cannot.)

The U.S. Supreme court also wrote that the scientists had added four plasmids to bacteria. Love found E. coli listed in most of the patents. These "modified" bacteria cannot be killed by antibiotics. [Other medical experts have commented that this has sinister applications in that these pathogens can possibly aid the spike proteins in embedding in and altering human DNA.]

Dr. Ariyana then explains, "They're snapping your DNA in half." A combo PCR COVID test (using hydrogels) also mentions "gene deletion." This is in addition to the Pfizer COVID vax patent, naming thirty gene deletions! A warning: interchanging XY chromosomes can cause sterility. Another study Love mentions found the sixty-nine to seventy gene deletions cause a variant that is significantly more transmissible [Omicron, anyone?]. Pfizer mentions gene #144. [This deletion is said by various COVID medical researchers to be linked with rapid cancer growth.]

Love tells us that Dr. Anthony Fauci owns the patent for "HIV that is in Moderna and J&J bioweapons." She explains, "Lentivirus is in Moderna and J&J, and other harmful COVID vaccine ingredients include bromide (Pfizer and Moderna). Pfizer mentions use of propane. Bromide is a corrosive that causes severe eye damage. Propane is an ingredient that is poisonous when inhaled. It is flammable and can be lethal. It will displace the oxygen in your lungs, making it hard to breathe, and now we're injecting it into our kids."

Dr. Ariyana Love believes that later, when millions around the world wake up, their fierce anger will bring the new Nuremberg Trials. [Editor's note: As late as July 23, 2021, NIH head Dr. Francis Collins was still out visiting churches, urging on COVID vaccinations. In a Baptist News Global interview, he said, "Give God the glory, but roll up your sleeve."]

— *Elizabeth Cuppett Caverly*

CHAPTER NINE

Part Two: Man Becoming A.I.?

INSIDE THE COVID VACCINE VIALS, SELF-AWARE ENTITIES? ... OPERATING SYSTEMS AND SUPER CONDUCTORS

Dr. Carrie Madej, Specialist—Internal Medicine, and Christian, conducted her first interview with Health Ranger Mike Adams in May 2021.

(Ethan Huff, NaturalNews.com, May 11. 2021)

> What seems to worry Dr. Madej the most is the synthetic components of Chinese Virus injections that basically turn humans into genetically modified organisms. What Big Pharma is doing by injecting messenger RNA (mRNA) components into people's bodies is transforming the human genome into something synthetic, rendering recipients as non-human chimeras.

Madej's warning words were: "They are putting synthetic genes, synthesized genes, and genomes inside of you. Is that human anymore? What does that to us?"

She discussed the harm COVID spike proteins in the injections do to the body, programming it to "hurt itself." Madej revealed the shocking truth that the Supreme Court agrees that it is entirely possible to patent humans and then turn them into the property of pharmaceutical companies through these types of injections, which, Madej explained, contain "exotic nanobots and other futuristic tech. Once these little particles get inside you, they can be used as processors. Could they be transmitting a signal or some kind of impulse to control you through outside stimuli, such as 5-G radiation?"

Dr. Madej asked, "What is wrong with our world right now? No human should be owned like a piece of property or chattel."

DR. CARRIE MADEJ, IN A LATER INTERVIEW, TOLD OF HER FAITH AND "SELF-AWARE" ENTITY

(Early 2022:) Stalwart heroine Dr. Carrie Madej's recent interview at Bitchute.com recounted how, years back, she first attended a meeting of what she thought was a typical medical industry progress-planning session. Instead, she was amazed to be witnessing the inception of plans that have now materialized in the cyborg-making messenger RNA COVID shots. Courage and belief in Jesus Christ are hallmarks of Carrie Madej's background. After her shocking discoveries at the planning meeting, God gave Carrie Madej wisdom to hide away in another country for five years! During that time, many of her peers back home died mysterious deaths. Indeed, even now, about two years ago, Madej and her fiancé were involved in a strange plane crash but were protected by God from death. And earlier, God brought her forth safely to 2021 when she could investigate COVID vaccines and expose the truth.

Next, in a September 29, 2021 (Brighteon.com) interview, Dr. Madej told how God had once more opened an unusual door of discovery. At the end of one day in a Georgia lab, the last person was injected with a Moderna vaccine, and Dr. Madej and others were legally able to examine under the microscope the leftover contents of the vial that would have been discarded.

In that Moderna vial, Dr. Madej observed a weird tentacle-like structure. This "creature" amazingly seemed to demonstrate "self-awareness." Madej described how it moved out to the edge of the microscope slide and seemed to lift itself off the slide! "We looked at this phenomenon that was under magnification (400×). This resembled a flying, dark angel. It also looked a lot like some pictures of Baphomet," she recalled.

Dr. Madej also saw colors strangely beginning to emerge in the vial. The substances in the Moderna vial were first colorless, then they transformed into brilliant blues, yellows, and purples. Another vial, this time a Johnson and Johnson sample, had fluorescent pastels. In J & J, Madej saw gray squares, graphene-like structures, spheres and rings. How could these colors emerge without a chemical reaction? When Dr. Madej questioned experts, she found that such colors are produced when white light (from the microscope) is shone on a superconducting material. What is this superconducting material? Carrie Madej's bombshell answer: "A superconductor is ***an injected operating system!***"

Moderna's mRNA operating system is perhaps revealing itself as an artificial intelligence tool. It may be one that will change, and keep changing, the bodies (and perhaps souls) of all the world's hapless men, women, and children who get jabbed. That goes for Pfizer, too. And what about Johnson and Johnson? Have we been lied to? We were told mRNA was not part of Johnson and Johnson's COVID vaccine. (Then how do Carrie Madej and the other Georgia lab workers also see structures apparently built by operating systems and bright colors in the J & J jabs?)

The Moderna "self-aware" entity that lifted itself up on the edge of the slide may be not be just a physical creation. It is perhaps a manifestation of supernatural evil—a symbol or perhaps a real force that can rob the souls of people. Those who willfully choose to put aborted fetal cell line-derived COVID vaccines [abomination to God] into their bodies.

In contrast, what about those unfortunate people (some of them our close friends and relatives), who did not know about or understand this anathema to God? They may possibly be forgiven by God's mercy. They may die a death that is sudden and perhaps even painless. It is possible that a fortunate few may have even been blessed to get some of the COVID vaccines that were, we understand, saline shots.

Is graphene oxide in the COVID vaccines? Many corroborations for this being true exist—from the writings of Archbishop Carlo Maria Vigano to Japan's scientific findings—all stating that graphene oxide has been found in the vaccines, with graphene oxide facilitating this hydrogel tubular nightmare. We seem to be entering the threshold of a not-so-brave new A.I. World.

Dr. Madej said these COVID vaccine analyses are proof they are putting an operating system inside people. This happened in the Moderna and Johnson and Johnson samples we observed. It is the beginning or advent of transhumanism. "This is **your** beginning, the advent to have surveillance and spying done on people" [emphasis added].

> Just like Bill Gates said he is doing in West Africa. People need to remember that the Gates Foundation or at least Bill Gates and GABI, his company, is working with MasterCard and Trust Stamp, an artificial intelligence program, testing it on people in West Africa, with their COVID vaccines, injections I should say, giving them a digital ID. They can only get their monetary funds through the digital ID and MasterCard, no other way—no cash, nothing; and all their medical records downloaded into this digital format in their body. And they said in this program (this research experiment they're doing on the people, the substance inside of them—this hydrogel substance, of course.) 'Why don't we use it for surveillance and predictive policing? We are going to use it on the people of West Africa right now' [emphasis added]. They've been administering the program since July of 2020.

Carrie Madej concluded, "*And they said that, once they have it perfected, they would like to unveil it in all the developed nations. They're calling it the Wellness Pass, which is also known as the vaccine passport. And how are they going to do that? They have to put something inside your body so they can know everything you're doing. ... We are children of God. I will not stand for it.*"

[Every Christian's true walk with God is being tested by the choice of being injected or not. We may be watching the "mark of the Beast" emerging in embryonic form. A vaccine passport is not a Christian's guide to life. Ours is not the wide way that leads to destruction and an eternal abode in hell. The living Word of God as found in the holy Scripture is our heavenly passport.

"Choose you this day whom ye will serve ..."

—Joshua 24:10

"There is a way which seemeth right unto a man,
but the end thereof are the ways of death."

—Proverbs 14:12

—Elizabeth Cuppett Caverly

CHAPTER TEN

Died Suddenly: "The Dead Doctor," "Maddy's Story and More"

The following story is very shocking:

Florida Man Develops and Dies from Rare Autoimmune Disorder Days after Receiving Pfizer Coronavirus Vaccine

(Arsenio Toledo, NaturalNews.com, January 25, 2021)
The Centers for Disease Control and Prevention (*CDC*), *the Florida Department of Health,* and the Miami-Dade County Medical Examiner Department are investigating the sudden passing of a doctor [https://humansarefree.com/2021/01/johns-hopkins-scientist-a-medical-certainty-pfizer-vaccine-caused-death-of-florida-doctor.html] who developed a rare autoimmune disorder several days after receiving Pfizer's coronavirus (COVID-19) vaccine.

Dr. Gregory Michael, a 56-year-old obstetrician and gynecologist from Miami Beach, received the vaccine [https://www.nytimes.com/2021/01/12/health/COVID-vaccine-death.html] at Mount Sinai Medical Center on Dec. 18. Just three days after receiving the vaccine, he developed a rare autoimmune disorder known as acute immune thrombocytopenia, which prevented his blood from clotting. On Jan. 3, his wife, Heidi Neckelmann, wrote in a Facebook post that he had died from a brain hemorrhage.

Pfizer almost immediately released a defensive statement saying there was no connection to the COVID-shot. Dr. Michael's wife said, too, he had absolutely no underlying medical condition.

> "He was an avid deep-sea fisherman and mostly a family man," she added. "He never got COVID because he used an N95 mask from the beginning of the pandemic. He was adamant in protecting his family and patients."
>
> Shortly after receiving the vaccine, Michael developed tiny spots called petechiae, which are formed when tiny blood vessels break open. Recognizing that something was wrong, Michael immediately went to the ER, where doctors discovered that his platelet count had gone down to zero. For two weeks, doctors tried to raise his platelet count, and medical experts from all over the world were involved in trying to save him.

This is very interesting because many of those medical experts knew Michael personally, were his friends and colleagues. *They wanted to save him!*

> Neckelmann shared the story that it "in this case" destroyed a beautiful life, a perfect family has affected so many people in the community."
>
> Dr. Lyn Redwood, president of Children's Health Defense, said that idiopathic thrombocytopenic purpura, the disorder that killed Michael, has been known to develop after inoculation with other vaccines.

THE STORY OF MADDIE

Both Great Game India (June 30, 2021) and NaturalNews.com (July 2, 2021) reported on this young girl's tragedy. The following excerpts are from the writer, Ethan Huff:

> **12-YEAR-OLD GIRL BOUND TO WHEELCHAIR WITH CHRONIC ILLNESS THANKS TO COVID VACCINE**
>
> Stephanie de Garay claims that her daughter Maddie was perfectly

> healthy before she and her brothers were enrolled in a Pfizer trial for children back in January. After receiving her second injection, young Maddie came down with a laundry list of horrific symptoms that have left her on an NG feeding tube.
>
> "Why is she not back to normal?" Stephanie asked as her daughter sat next to her and listened quietly.
>
> As you will notice in the above video clip, Maddie's facial reactions do not seem to align with what her mother is saying, suggesting that the child is now suffering from some kind of brain damage.
>
> Stephanie confirmed this, also indicating Maddie can no longer feel any body parts below her waist, hence why she is now bound to a wheelchair.

Great Game India also reported on the June 2021 press conference held with a few people who told their post-vaccine stories.

> Candace Hayden was one of six people who came to share their stories. Hayden says:
>
> *"We are asking to be seen, we're asking to be heard, and we are asking to be believed. I was suffering from severe paresthesia and was partially paralyzed from the chest down."*
>
> From shooting pain in their bodies to being unable to move, attendees recalled the dreadful moments of what their life has since turned into after getting their vaccinations.
>
> *"I lost control of my legs, and my bladder, along with my dignity,"* said one participant, Brianne Dressen.
>
> *"On Jan. 14, I received the Moderna vaccine. The next morning, I woke up with severely swollen lymph nodes in my neck,"* said another participant, Sheryl Ruetgers.

At the press conference, Sen. Ron Johnson stated he believes the CDC and other health officials aren't being "totally transparent." One might have thought this congressional photo op moment might begin to stop the gain of function research in its tracks. But no, TWO YEARS LATER we look back after perhaps a billion people have "died suddenly," and scorn Senator Johnson's lukewarm press conference statement:

> *"That small minority that are suffering severe symptoms, they want to deny that reality. I am not advocating anything other than to listen to these people and to take them seriously."*

[Editor's Note: Yes, it is so crucial having the etiquette to be a good listener.]

THREE MILESTONE 2021 HEADLINES

> "Pope Francis Calls for a New World Order inhabited by fully vaccinated slaves" (NaturalNews.com, April 15, 2021) [The pope sent this message to the spring 2021 meeting of the World Bank and the International Monetary Fund (IMF). In his letter he officially called for a new system of "global governance" and "universal vaccines."]

> "Bombshell: DARPA was secretly developing the mRNA vaccine years ago through Moderna and they seek permanent control over your body and bloodline." (NaturalNews.com, August 17, 2021)

> "Unvaccinated Americans refuse blood transfusion from vaccinated donors due to spike protein fears." (NaturalNews.com, August 23, 2021, Nolan Barton) [Dr. Michael Busch, Vilatent Research Institute director said more than 90 percent of current donors have either been infected with COVID-19 or vaccinated against it.]

Art Moore, on World Net Daily, September 30, 2021, spotlighted an unbelievable CDC headline. This malevolent suggestion, "CDC: 'Urgent for "pregnant people" to get COVID vaccine.'" Once my husband, Lou Caverly, looked at the CDC website and gasped, "Gosh, Elizabeth. Look at this! The CDC entrance gate looks just like a tombstone!" It did! Maybe this oddity was like a miniature Georgia Guidestones. A smaller

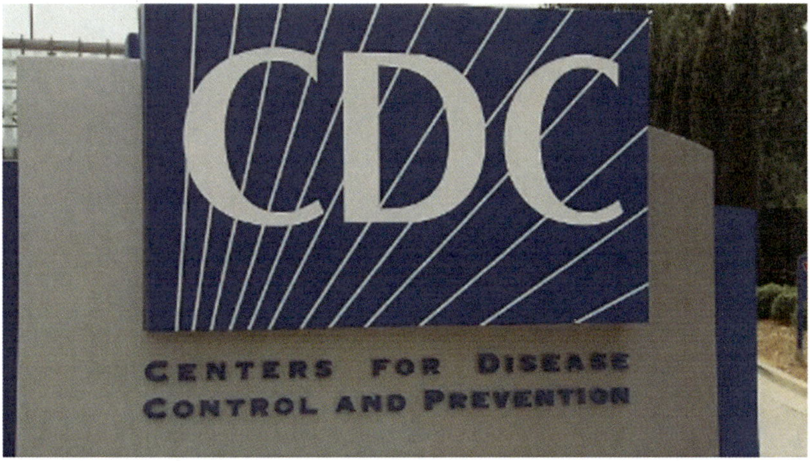

"depopulation marker." The CDC, you recall, gave us the PCR test. A test that they, themselves, later condemned as not accurate. During lockdowns, the strangely powerful CDC was even able to issue edicts to prevent landlords from evicting renters.

We also recall that, in the early COVID days, Fox News reported about two college girls returning from Italy. Since Italy was a COVID hotbed at that time, the girls conscientiously stopped in New York before heading to their homes in the South. Not wanting to spread COVID, they called the CDC and inquired, "Should we quarantine?" The CDC advised, "No, girls. Just run along home!" One has to wonder whether the CDC is there, not to control disease, but to spread it.

Its Jesuit connections are worth noting. Interestingly, the institution's founder attended Marquette, the Jesuit research university, in the early 1900s. In a recent 2023 Divided Kingdom radio interview, documentary filmmaker Christian J. Pinto alluded to the apparent political and medical "Jesuit stronghold" connection in the unconstitutional coup we seem to be in since the "stolen" 2020 election. Pinto noted the strongly Jesuit-educated Anthony Fauci and President Joe Biden.

By fall, 2021, pregnant women who listened to the CDC's vaccine advice were counterpunched. A Natural News headline from November 23 (writer Ethan Huff) reads, "Whistleblowers expose 13 stillborn deaths in 24 hours at Lion's Gate Hospital [British Columbia] caused by COVID 'vaccines.'"

The video "Died Suddenly" went viral worldwide, but the post-COVID vaccine deaths kept happening and the timed "depopulation sudden deaths" are still occurring.

As we conclude writing this book, in late summer 2023, here is a fresh portrait of tragedy. It is not verified whether this unfortunate young girl had had the COVID "vaccine." One would suppose it likely, because of her father's executive J&J position. *When will God's church leaders in America ever shout, "ENOUGH"?*

> July 5, 2023—Princeton, NJ—**10-year-old Kelsey Morand, daughter of J&J COVID-19 Vaccine Executive Mike Morand, died suddenly from a seizure**
>
> A tragic incident unfolded earlier this month when the young daughter of a Johnson & Johnson COVID-19 vaccine executive died suddenly from a bout of seizures. According to her family, 10-year-old Kelsey Corinne Morand suffered a fatal brain injury following a seizure on July 3. She began having seizures on July 1 and flatlined for 20 minutes, she was intubated, and continued having seizures and died July 5.

—*Elizabeth Cuppett Caverly*

CHAPTER ELEVEN

Part Three: Behind the Clot Shot Oz Curtain: Turning Us Into "The Tin Man"

Dr. Zandré Botha, PhD in alternative medicine, has her practice in South Africa. A guest on the "Stew Peters Show," October 4, 2021, Dr. Botha explained how she had examined blood taken from non-vaccinated patients and compared it with blood from persons who had been vaccinated. She showed slides of both samples. The comparison was shocking. Just as could be seen earlier in similar slides that Dr. Jane Ruby showed from UK's Dr. Wellburn, the blood of unvaccinated patients had normal, round, red blood cells uniformly spaced and not clumped. In the blood of those who had been vaccinated, the red blood cells were clumped, distorted, and appeared to be sticking together. Botha remarked that these injured cells would not be able to deliver oxygen effectively. They would have a very hard time passing through the smaller capillaries. These slides were shocking enough. But the strangest were yet to come.

Dr. Botha described in looking at her microscope slide-findings, that she first saw some irregular-shaped dark "blobs." Next to appear were black metal disks joined to each other by some type of "metal" connectors. She commented on this very distinctive phenomenon. "They look engineered; they look very symmetrical."

These disks were arranged in consistent patterns, in several instances having six situated around and practically tangent to a central disk. Also, the very short "bonds" joining the disks were equally spaced around the central disk. This would maximize the available space. As most of us may recall from geometry class, exactly six circles can surround and be tangential to a single circle of the same size. Dr. Botha said they were "too structured to be biological." (This would infer that these "rings" belonged more to the world of artificial intelligence than to the world of humanity.)

In her fifteen years of work, this doctor has never seen anything like this. When asked by Dr. Botha, many fellow physicians told her she was not seeing "air bubbles." They said, "Air bubbles do not have such symmetry in their arrangement. Nor are they attached to each other by 'bonds.'"

Dr. Botha found another amazing occurrence after leaving the vaccine sample out in the air. The disks had completely disappeared! In their place were satanic-looking jagged lines. They resembled a barbed-wire fence—almost like the razor wire once at the Capitol! Some of them were almost perfectly parallel to each other for part of their length. They reminded us of a medieval torture device or a jagged-toothed spring trap used to catch small animals. ***Who's being caught in this witches' brew concoction?***

These "construction" lines form a network in which any point can be reached from another by following some combination of the lines. They reminded me of a schematic diagram of a complex electrical circuit. Is it possible that in some way they serve this function? Perhaps to transmit information to a surveillance source outside the body? Or to permit someone on the outside to maneuver what goes on within the body? The 5-G scenario possibility for control of the masses comes to mind.

Dr. Zandré Botha is treating many patients who have been vaccinated. She described the illnesses they have suffered post "clot" shot. Severe embolisms, memory loss, blood clots, loss of movement at the injection site, nerve pain, and shortness of breath. They are breathless because the oxygen levels in their blood are very low since the mangled red blood cells are unable to do their job. White blood cells are also affected.

Dr. Botha weeps, just as did Dr. Carrie Madej, when she sees some of her COVID-injured patients actually plan to take their **children** to get the shots! One man, her incoming patient, had eight heart attacks in five hours. He had been chosen as a "guinea pig" for the COVID vaccine roll-out. He has been in the ICU for months since March. This man could not get a triple bypass because he kept testing positive for COVID. His life is being controlled by a "vicious circle" of revolving positive COVID tests.

The mRNA "operating system" inside the vaccine—with its sinister maze of bioengineered lines—symbolizes not just vaccine tyranny to this one man. No, there may ultimately be millions now living under severe chronic illness and injury. Or not living at all—cut off by sudden death.

My wife asked, "Who would have thought in our lifetime that people could be tricked into becoming half-machines?" She then murmured, "Why it's 'Behind the Clot-Shot Oz Curtain, Turning us into The Tin Man!'" And so, my title for this article was born.

—*Lou Caverly*

CHAPTER TWELVE

Died Suddenly: Top World Athletes

As early as November 10, 2021, Lance Johnson at NaturalNews.com wrote this headline and the subsequent article we excerpt:

> **The world is starting to notice how many young athletes are DYING after taking COVID vaccines**
>
> A German newspaper, *Berliner Zeitung*, took note of this disturbing pattern of cardiac arrest in a report titled, "Puzzling heart diseases in football." The report seeks to understand why an "unusually large number of professional and amateur soccer players have collapsed recently." The world is starting to notice how many young athletes are suffering and DYING after taking COVID vaccines. Jake Kazmarek, a 28-year-old bodybuilder died unexpectedly four days after taking a COVID vaccine. Another recently vaccinated athlete collapsed in the middle of a game; hockey player Boris Sadecky (24) died after suddenly collapsing on the ice.
>
> Young athletes who aren't at risk from a natural infection are continuously being coerced to take experimental mRNA spike protein vaccines in order to keep their careers. The spike protein encoded in people's cells was designed to kill red blood cells by hampering their ability to transport oxygen. The spike proteins have also been shown to cause clumping in the blood, leading to blood clots. Dr. Richard Fleming demonstrates a nefarious characteristic of the Pfizer vaccine, by showing microscopically how red blood cells are deprived

> of oxygen when they are contacted by the vaccine ingredients. As Dr. Judy Mikovits points out, these spike proteins were designed in a lab with a component from HIV. They also contain syncytin, allowing the vaccine to express cancer genes, and cause reproductive harm and immunodeficiency. Even the *Wall Street Journal* is now commenting on the damage done by these vaccines, which includes heart inflammation, pericarditis, and myocarditis.

Mark Playne from "Not on the Been" has been keeping a running list of professional sports players who develop sudden health issues, including death, almost immediately after getting injected for the Fauci Flu. The following are some of the cases he had documented by November 13, 2021:

- » Lexi Riggles, a college basketball player who "died unexpectedly" back in October
- » Tom Greenway, a champion jockey who died in early November
- » Nelson Solano, a Spanish footballer who died of a heart attack in early November
- » Shawn Rhoden, a bodybuilder and former Mr. Olympia who died of an apparent heart attack in early November
- » Layla da Costa, a Miss World contestant from Italy who was found dead at her house after failing to show up for work
- » George "Da Bull" Peterson III, who was found dead in a Florida hotel room just two days before he was scheduled to compete in the Mr. Olympia contest
- » Jordan Tucker, a footballer who passed away unexpectedly during play
- » Avi Barot, a Saurashtra batter who died after suffering cardiac arrest

From National File, September 30, 2022 by Frankie Stokes:

> **16-Year-Old Boy Drops Dead After Taking Pfizer Jab**
>
> An American teenager dropped dead just five days after taking the

Pfizer jab while he was running onto the basketball court to play with a friend.

16-year-old Texan Ernesto Ramirez died in April of 2021, just five days after taking the Pfizer jab, with doctors blaming the heart condition of myocarditis for his sudden demise—the calling card of COVID jab deaths.

Since then, Ernesto's father Ernest has channeled his grief to travel the country raising awareness and protecting other kids from the lethal side effects of experimental COVID jabs.

A Jaw-Dropping 769 Athletes Have Collapsed While Competing Over the Past Year

(Julian Conradson, The Gateway Pundit, April 8, 2022)

Over the past year-plus, athletes across the world have been dropping like flies as they compete in games. If they aren't passed out cold, they are seen gripping their chests in agony, unable to breathe due to sudden cardiac events that hit in the heat of the competition.

This wave of heart issues is unprecedented, to say the least. Never before have we seen young, healthy, world-class athletes experiencing heart issues en masse like this. It has never happened, ever.

COVID is not over! No, it's still a part of the "coming chaos" in our book's title. The timed-release spike protein in "sudden deaths" and/or severe injuries are still happening. How many more will come, even in 2025?

IT'S STILL HAPPENING! HEAT OF A *DEADLY* SUMMER

July 2023 Sports Soundbites—Lou Caverly

» Infowars, July 24, 2023 reported: An ESPN analyst collapsed live on-air Sunday during a soccer pre-game show, prompting his co-anchor to call for help as he attempted to aid his fellow broadcaster. ESPN host Dan Thomas was talking to anchor and former soccer player **Shaka Hislop,** 54, when Hislop's knees started to buckle and he suddenly stumbled onto the floor. [Hislop had "heavily promoted" the COVID vaccination.]

- Late July 2023—all over the news came the story of **Bronny James**'s sudden emergency. The AP, July 28 said: The Los Angeles Lakers superstar LeBron James's 18-year-old son, Bronny, was hospitalized Monday morning after a basketball practice with his team at the University of Southern California. He was hospitalized at Cedars-Sinai Medical Center, where he was in stable condition Tuesday.
- The Gateway Pundit, July 7, 2023, by Jim Hoft: "On Friday, **Edwin van der Sar**, Manchester United legend and former Netherlands International goalkeeper, was admitted to the Intensive Care Unit (ICU) in Croatia following an unexpected brain hemorrhage. ... On June 1, 2021, Van der Sar announced that he had received his COVID-19 vaccine."
- The Gateway Pundit, July 28, 2023, reported: "22-year-old ex-Premier League Star Forced to Retire Early Due to Myocarditis." **Lars Dendoncker** was the incapacitated "footballer."
- ThePeoplesVoice.tv, July 5, 2023, stated: "UFC fighter **Anthony 'Lionheart' Smith** has publicly revealed that the COVID-19 vaccination not only killed his mother but also left him with potentially deadly blood clots."
- Outkick.com, July 21, 2023, had the lamentable story of well-known wide receiver **Marquise Goodwin**: "Goodwin has blood clots in his legs and lungs, the Cleveland Browns announced Friday. The veteran wide receiver said he began feeling discomfort in his legs and shortness of breath during team workouts this spring. A check-up revealed the clots."
- The Gateway Pundit, July 7, 2023, had this headline by writer Cullen Linebarger: "17-Year-Old New York Football Player in Coma after Collapsing on the Field Due to 'Cardiac Event'—Had No Known Heart Problems ... **Robert Bush** was undergoing conditioning drills ... when he suddenly bent over and passed out ... His brother, Steve, said, 'There's no more brain function.

We are dealing with the end right now.'"

» LifeSite News, July 7, 2023, showed this headline: "Canadian dad says US doctor confirmed his 17-year-old son was killed by the COVID vaccine ... **Sean Hartman** of New Tecumseth, Ontario, died at home of a heart attack only 33 days after getting his first Pfizer COVID-19 injection. American pathologist Dr. Ryan Cole confirmed [he] died from the COVID shot after finding evidence of spike proteins present in his adrenal glands."

CHAPTER THIRTEEN

Part Four: Still More Evidence of A.I. Mechanisms in COVID Vaccines

LifeSite News had the following excellent in-depth coverage of Dr. Nixon's research and Matt Taylor's findings:

Australian Doctor Finds Chips, 'Self-Assembling' Structures Forming in Pfizer Vaccine Contents

(Emily Mangiaracina, LifeSite News, December 2, 2022)

An Australian doctor has gone public with microscopic images of unidentified objects that appear to be "self-assembling" from the contents of Pfizer's COVID injection.

Family physician Dr. David Nixon recently shared dark field microscopy photos of "concerning" structures that appeared in Pfizer jab fluid over time and that seem to be the product of "intelligent design" in a Sunday episode of the International Crimes Investigative Committee (ICIC) co-hosted by the group's founder, Dr. Reiner Fuellmich and ex-Pfizer executive Dr. Michael Yeadon.

Nixon showed how boxy, dark structures, similar in shape to crystals but with "internal structures that appear to be different from ... a naturally occurring crystal," appeared on the periphery of the slide's jab contents after he left it out overnight.

Remarkably, the formation of the crystalline structures appeared to depend on their exposure to electromagnetic frequencies (EMFs), according to Nixon. When he put the slide "inside a faraday bag" blocking EMFs he said came from his wireless router, he only saw black, round "dots."

However, when he "didn't shield the site," only the angular, crystal-like formations "would appear the next morning."

The LifeSite article also mentioned that other reports have come in about EMFs affecting structure formations in the COVID jab fluid:

> Electrical engineer Matt Taylor in Ecuador testified on a Brighteon.com radio show that when he put a drop of the COVID jab on a microscope slide and placed that slide on an internet router, he observed the self-assembly of what he believes "look like integrated circuits." When Taylor turned the router off, the objects "immediately" began to break apart. He repeated the experiment three times and "begged" people to reproduce his investigation to see if his findings can be replicated. In fact, Nixon indicated that Taylor had inspired his own test with the faraday bag.
>
> Nixon's experimental study showed that when the COVID fluid was left out in the open, on the slide (for ten weeks), something strange happened. The crystalline shapes morphed, taking on "the appearance of a much more concerning nature." Those structures Nixon showed maintained angular shapes, but now appeared to contain one or more bright light-reflecting points, in addition to other interior formations. The close-ups of these objects were photographed at 200x magnification, Nixon told LifeSiteNews. The structures, which Nixon now called "chips," had moved from being present, not only on the periphery of the slide's jab contents, but to being all throughout it. Nixon shared with LifeSiteNews a video running at 200x speed that highlighted both relatively small and large lights that seemed to suddenly appear in the "chip."
>
> These chips were also "often associated with" new ribbon-like objects that Nixon now describes as "wires"—that is, they often appeared alongside the "wires." Nixon said that he has seen similar "wire" formations in the blood of the vaccinated. He showed LifeSite

> News a picture in which clumping blood cells surround the "wire" with "frayed edges," that Nixon says are often present.
>
> The article told how two electrical engineers—Yanowitz and Taylor—have an interesting conclusion about what they have observed in COVID vaccine fluid under the microscope. They have seen what strongly resemble electronic "circuits." Others, too, have told about finding of "self-assembling" jab structures.

The LifeSite News article mentions other key researchers' findings: Dr. Carrie Madej first observed what she referred to as the "self-assembling" of unidentified objects specifically in the Moderna injection.

By contrast, in the Pfizer jab, Madej observed "something that looks similar to teslaphoresis," which, she explains, is "when these little graphite-like black, metallic particles start to coalesce into strings, like a spider web. They do that through any external force—it could be light, it could be a magnetic force, it could be an impulse, like a frequency."

Karen Kingston, who used to do marketing work for Pfizer, pointed out that "80 percent" of the "ingredients, the manufacturing process, and the toxicity" of the COVID jabs was "redacted under the FDA law since it was approved. We have the right under FOIA (Freedom of Information Act) to know what those ingredients are. These are not biologics," Kingston said.

—*Elizabeth Cuppett Caverly*

CHAPTER FOURTEEN

Died Suddenly: Celebrity Casualties

Some of America's best-loved celebrities sadly perished during "Operation Warp Speed." Bob Saget, the popular TV father in the beloved "Full House" series was one of the first notable casualties. Here is an excerpt from NaturalNews.com editors, January 10, 2022 (article by Kelen McBreen, republished from Infowars.com):

> The Orange County Florida Sheriff's Office announced on Twitter Sunday that legendary comedian and actor Bob Saget was found dead in his hotel room at age 65. "Earlier today, deputies were called to the Ritz-Carlton Orlando, Grande Lakes for a call about an unresponsive man in a hotel room," the post stated. "The man was identified as Robert Saget and pronounced deceased on scene. Detectives found no signs of foul play or drug use in this case."
>
> Notably, Saget admitted during a December 13 episode of his podcast "Bob Saget's Here For You" that he had received a COVID booster jab just days before. "I went to the pharmacy the other day and got a booster shot," he explained. "I should have gotten it in my arm, but I got it in my butt. I try not to preach. I got my booster shot. I got my booster shot the day before yesterday," Saget said towards the end of the podcast.
>
> On November 28, the comedian posted a joke about the booster shot on Twitter. Throughout the pandemic, Saget frequently promoted the experimental mRNA shots on social media. In a February Twitter

post, the "Full House" star insinuated the COVID vaccines would eliminate COVID by 2023.

In May, the comedian talked with CBS News about vaccine hesitancy and "real facts" about the vaccine. A post from August declaring, "I don't wanna preach," went on to ask followers to "please get your vaccine today," claiming they "save lives." The vaccine appeared to be a huge joke to Saget, who once jested that he gets vaccinated "five to six times a day" and still feels great.

"We are devastated to confirm that our beloved Bob passed away," Saget's family said in a statement.

Two weeks ago, a *New York Times* editor died from an unexpected heart attack just one day after he received the Moderna COVID-19 booster vaccine. Meanwhile, as mainstream media ignores the data and Big Tech silences any dissenting viewpoints online. A report from the UK Health Security Agency reveals vaccinated people made up nearly 75% of COVID-19 deaths in Britain from Dec. 6 to Jan. 2.

The COVID Death Syndrome did not end when "Operation Warp Speed" concluded. In 2023 (and no doubt 2024 and 2025) the mRNA "timed life-termination model" will continue to depopulate. During 2023 we have learned that Elon Musk was another famous figure harmed.

(David McLoome, LifeSiteNews, January 21, 2023)

Billionaire entrepreneur and Twitter owner Elon Musk announced that he had "major side effects" after taking his "second booster shot" of the COVID jabs. The illness he experienced after the booster left him wondering if he would suffer "permanent damage" from the injection.

In a tweet shared Saturday morning, the Tesla and SpaceX founder shared that following reception of his "second booster" he "felt like [he] was dying for several days," before adding a hopeful note that no "permanent damage" may have been caused.

Musk later added that his cousin, "who is young and in peak health, had a serious case of myocarditis" following inoculation, leading to his hospitalization. Indeed, so-called vaccine-induced myocarditis has been indicated in a growing number of cases of sudden deaths, often in young and athletic men, from around the world.

"This SARS-CoV-2 outbreak was bad enough as it is, but now the mass vaccination program, which has been administered to two-thirds of the world's population, has been a debacle," Dr. Peter McCullough said in comments to LifeSiteNews. "Recall that we had COVID-19 in 2020 for the full year, and there really wasn't an increase in all-cause mortality. But it really ticked up in 2021 and 2022. Skyrocketed, in fact. And the only new exposure now is mass vaccination. We're seeing it across the world recently."

McCullough also suggested that 37-year old Oklahoma country singer Jake Flint, who died suddenly in his sleep in November last year, might have been a victim of the jab. "The working diagnosis is that it's subclinical vaccine-induced myocarditis," he said. In light of the uptick in "sudden adult death syndrome" blamed for the unprecedented hike in numbers of young men suffering fatal cardiac arrests, McCullough argued that vaccine-induced myocarditis, as a result of COVID inoculation, ought to be presumed. Responding to Musk's tweet Saturday, McCullough said that his adverse reaction to the COVID booster is a case of "reactogenicity," which he stated increases from the first to the second jab by 80 times, and increases further by the third shot.

Elvis Pressley's beloved daughter, Lisa Marie, sadly became the next casualty.

(Meredith Nardino, *US Magazine,* "Austin Butler Reacts to Lisa Presley's Death After Elvis' Biopic: 'My Heart Is Completely Shattered,'" January 13, 2023)

Always on his mind. "I am eternally grateful for the time I was lucky enough to be near her bright light and will forever cherish the quiet moments we shared. Her warmth, her love and her authenticity will always be remembered."

Us Weekly confirmed on Thursday, January 12, that the Tennessee native was hospitalized after going into ***cardiac arrest.*** Hours later, her mother, Priscilla Presley, announced that Lisa Marie died at age 54. "It is with a heavy heart that I must share the devastating news that my beautiful daughter Lisa Marie has left us," the 77-year-old, who was married to Elvis Presley from 1967 to 1973, told *People* in a statement.

Very strangely, "revisionist" reports have just emerged in summer 2023 that Lisa Marie died from some kind of "blockage." What happened to the earlier reports, including *US Magazine's* that authenticated Lisa Marie's "emergency situation" was a ***cardiac arrest?*** Is there some kind of cover-up for still another post-COVID vaccine death? Money and power throughout time have always been able to obscure the truth.

Also odd, we thought, was that no circumstances or cause was listed for legendary comedian Betty White's death. She was in her nineties, but had remained active and vibrant. Why was there no information about what triggered her passing away?

Mysterious, just as the obituary of a young eight-year-old in our Maryland newspaper. No facts, no details. Was it another "died suddenly"?

How about mega-star Jamie Foxx? What was the early shocking report concerning a sudden stroke emergency?

> Brighteon.com's Dr. Jane Ruby said, Foxx is just the latest [among] the ... scores of pro-jab celebrities taking a hit to their health after self-righteously promoting the jab," she said during the April 17 episode of the Brighteon.TV program "Dr. Jane Ruby STAT!"
>
> According to her, the latest news out of Hollywood is that the fully vaccinated actor of *Ray* and *Django Unchained* fame recently suffered a stroke that led to his hospitalization.

Let's examine the fact of Jamie Foxx's pro-vaccine statements and stance. Was it an isolated instance among Hollywood celebrities? The April 21, 2023, NaturalNews article (by Kevin Hughes) answers that question:

> Other pro-vaccine celebrities that suffered vaccine injuries include Australian actor Hugh Jackman of *The Greatest Showman* and *Van Helsing* fame, who suffered from skin cancer. Canadian singer Justin Bieber, known for his songs "Baby" and "Sorry," suffered facial paralysis due to the COVID-19 vaccine. (Related: Justin Bieber's face paralyzed with Ramsay Hunt syndrome, a known adverse reaction of COVID injections.)

People magazine brings us up to date on the latest Jamie Foxx news. In May and June, we had heard that Foxx, having begun rehabilitation, was still having difficulty walking. The July 17, 2023, issue of *People* states, "Jamie Foxx 'Still Not Himself' After Health Crisis":

> Three months after being hospitalized for an undisclosed medical complication, Jamie Foxx's recovery continues. "He is getting the best care and working hard to recover, but he is still not himself," a source says of the 55-year-old actor.

Late summer 2023. We are nearing the end of writing this book, *COVID and Coming Chaos.* We lament, as do all of you, the fact that some of our friends and family died suddenly (or were injured) after the COVID-19 shots. Celebrities entertain us, but *REAL PEOPLE WHO MATTER MOST TO US IN OUR EVERYDAY LIVES CAUSE US THE MOST PAIN WHEN THEY, LIKE INNOCENT LAMBS, GO TO THE SLAUGHTER. WITH NO WARNINGS WHATSOEVER FROM A DEAD CHURCH IN AMERICA.*

Lou and I, in our weekly "News Blitz" segment on DividedKingdomRadio.com, will keep warning, politically and spiritually—as events move us further—deeper into the ***coming chaos.*** *THERE IS ALWAYS HOPE—AND VICTORY—IN JESUS CHRIST!*

—*Elizabeth Cuppett Caverly*

CHAPTER FIFTEEN

Part Five: Transhumanism—Turning You Into a Machine—Trackable, Traceable

Karen Kingston, on the "Stew Peters Show," September 22, 20022, commented:

Transhumanism or A.I. will "transform, track and subjugate mankind." Shocking new driver of this anti-human crusade is the newly signed Joe Biden executive order, "Advancing Biotechnology and Bio-Manufacturing Innovation for Sustainable, Safe and Secure American Bioeconomy." Stew Peters warned, "This is advancing (1) trans-humanism and (2) the use of genetic engineering to make us less human and more machine ..." Kingston completed his thought, "... and to make us more ***controllable***." She added, "COVID injections were nothing more than electronic surveillance under the skin and enslavement. ..."

The statement released by Biden is highly disturbing:

> We need to develop genetic technologies and techniques to be able to write circuitry for cells and predictably program biology in the same way in which we write software and program computers; unlock the power of biological data, including through computing tools and artificial intelligence and advance the science of scale-up production while reducing the obstacles for commercialization so the innovative technologies and products can reach markets faster.

Kingston summarized the intent of "Transhumanism" to "augment the functionality of humans" (1) using biotechnology, (2) *genetic editing,* (3) these in combination with super-computers. She reiterated this nanotechnology's purpose was to hook humans up to the internet.

Nature magazine, August 2022, documents the imminent launch of the computer system, "Cubic Quantum," that will accumulate and analyze data. Kingston prognosticated that, "Then they can unleash Star Link and 5-G in order to send the signals to and from the technology to achieve the Biden 'societal goals.'" She added parenthetically that these societal goals are World Economic Forum goals to ***enslave***. Also, Biden's eerie executive order listed all the departments of the U.S. government that are part of this—working hand-in-hand with international organizations. Using the following data: (1) genomic information; (2) tracked info; (3) *record of your INTERACTIONS WITH OTHER PEOPLE*—These could be used to go after dissidents, even kill them.

Ominously, Biden's very words reveal the future "Frankenstein" goal of the Joint Artificial Intelligence Center. "Their mission is to (1) *allow de-centralized EXECUTION AND EXPERIMENTATION"*; (2) *"accelerate delivery of A.I. throughout society"*; and (3) "partner with corporations throughout society." Dr. Lynne Parker, head of the White House Task Force for A.I. (director of the National Artificial Intelligence Initiative Office) concurred with these points when the Organization for Economic Cooperation and Development met, Kingston reiterated. *"TO TRANSFORM IS THE GOAL OF A.I."*

You say, "America will never be part of this." Karen Kingston shocks us that *THIS INFORMATION IS RIGHT IN THE CURES ACT AND THERE ON THE DoD. WEBSITE!* Biden actually said (September 11, 2022, in his "Moon Shot Talk" at the Kennedy Center), that "he was elected President to do this." The ***"this"*** to be accomplished requires a lot of money delineated by Biden as follows:

- » $1.5 ***billion*** to Precise Medicine [to track and trace everyone]
- » $1.5 ***billion*** to DARPA (Defense Advanced Research Projects Agency) for the BRAIN INITIATIVE (neuro implants under the

> brain that can be delivered by small injection and then connected to an external server for signal exchange.

Kingston summed up this horrific "Brain Initiative": "Now our government is letting us know the plan they have for the American people. ***You'll be a machine and you'll be controlled.***"

We recall once more that the late documentary filmmaker Aaron Russo once told Alex Jones on air that his one-time close friend Nick Rockefeller confided in him that the top globalists' goal was to get a brain chip in every person on Earth. Lou Caverly and I have written this book to make you aware; to take action to save yourself; and most of all, to "stand in the gap," trust that Jesus Christ will guide, guard and, at last, save you in His eternal kingdom.

"METROPOLIS" A.I. TYRANNY COMING

November 2, 2021

Lou Caverly had two essays in October 2021 describing the microscope findings of Dr. Carrie Madej and Dr. Zandré Botha: circular chains of metal disks symmetrically arranged in a liquid sea. This appeared to be a "payload" system. What was being delivered? Why would the admitted mRNA "operating system" need these accouterments in the so-called "COVID vaccines"?

Another mystery is why some COVID vaccine recipients find they have "glowing" fingers or hands. Wednesday, October 27, Stew Peters interviewed "Amanda," a military wife, unidentified for obvious reasons of protection. Her husband has been in the military for fifteen years. He was coerced, with the threat of court martial to finally take the COVID shot.

After the vaccination, Amanda's husband became extremely fatigued, had terrible headaches, and constantly felt a heavy weight on his chest. Seeking alternative help, the couple arranged for a metallic clay bath for detoxification purposes. The procedure brought forth:

1. Anguished pain during the "Morgellons' Cleanse" as metallic strings came out of his body. These were similar to the strange "organism" Dr. Carrie Madej saw lift itself on a microscope slide that she deemed ***"almost self-aware."*** The military man's wife watched ***one such "string" seemingly try to wiggle back into her husband's body.***
2. The doctor's report in a letter stated that he observed damaged white blood cells and metallic strings apparently "attached" to the endothelial cells—something that doctor never sees in the unvaccinated. The physician also expressed ***GRAVE CONCERN*** about all the ***micro-clots*** he could observe being formed.
3. The ex-military man's fingers "glowed" brightly.

What does this clinical picture of symptoms mean? Is it an embryonic A.I. supratyranny-tracking system, light years removed from the rudimentary control practices in the fictitious 1927 movie ***Metropolis?*** In that powerful, early silent film, worker-slaves were subjugated in a level below the city.

Ninety years after the initial screening of *Metropolis*, the CEO of Bill Gates' GAVI, Global Vaccine Alliance, wrote in *Nature* magazine, urging moving the masses into digital ID systems. Then, one year later, in 2018, GAVI made the announcement that digital identity was the focus of its INFUSE program. This correlated with goal 16.9 of U.N. Agenda 2030. (This new update of the former Agenda 21 goals appeared in September 2015 and was approved by 100 nations.)

A graphic at GAVI's website, later removed, laid out the final ominous stage of the digital-identity health passport system, called "Access to Other Services." An excerpt: ***"... The digital child health card can be used to access secondary services, such as primary school or financial services, serving as the foundation for a broadly recognized digital identity."***

LifeSiteNews writer Leo Hohmann comments Friday, October 29, 2021:

> So you see where they are going with this whole health passport scam. It has nothing to do with your health. Your physical, digital,

> and financial life will all be tied together into one nifty little digital identification card, scannable with a QR code on your cellphone. Is it a coincidence that starting in 2022, all of the older cell phones, flip phones, and 'burner phones' will be phased out, no longer serviceable by your cell service provider? Conform or get left behind; the decision is yours. As for me and mine, leaving it behind is starting to look better and better.

October 26, 2021, LifeSiteNews carried an extended warning with this shocking title: "Abp. Vigano warns US bishops about COVID jab: The Great Reset wants billions of chronically ill people." Diametrically at odds with Dr. Richard Fleming's dismissive statement about graphene oxide, Archbishop Vigano says:

> The presence of graphene in the doses that have been administered, reported by numerous laboratories that have analyzed its content, suggests that the forced use of so-called vaccines—together with the systematic boycott of existing treatments of proven effectiveness—***serves the purpose of contact-tracing all vaccinated human beings throughout the world, who will be or already are connected to the Internet of Things*** by means of a quantum link of pulsed microwave frequencies of 2.4 GHz or higher from cell towers and satellites. As proof that this information is not the fruit of the fantasies of some conspiracy theorist, you should know that the European Union has chosen two projects dedicated to technological innovation as the winners of a competition: "The Human Brain" and "Graphene." These two projects will receive one billion euros each in funding over the next ten years.

Former Pfizer worker Karen Kingston tells us more about the futuristic version of *Metropolis* we are facing. Not only does the Vatican have a telescopic apparatus named ***"Lucifer,"*** but Pfizer uses Bill Gates' "***Lucifer***ase," having some connection to or derivation from a firefly that "glows blue."

Kingston's interview evokes the biblical parallel of "The time of Noah," Jesus' warning of a time, as in the Nephilim "giants" era, when fallen angels had progeny with Earth women. Now we are seeing CRISPR edit DNA using mRNA "operating systems." She states (October 28, Stew Peters interview, Brighteon.com), *"THE WORLD PATENT, MASTER PATENT ON mRNA, TABLE 54 AT THE MODERNA WEBSITE, STATES THE VACCINE CONTAINS LUCIFERASE FOR 'HYBRIDIZATION.'"* ***HYBRIDIZATION!***

Dr. Ariyana Love's October 28, 2022, interview offers corroboration. According to Dr. Love, there ARE hydras in the vaccine that have been genetically modified in a lab at the University of Kiev. They have been "transfected." Love studied NIH and DARPA open-source documents, reaching the conclusion these fresh water organisms surviving in the blood are there to "transfect" humans using the Lente virus. The research, she says, has gone on at Mars Hill and other places. The hydra and parasite's codes are being fused with the human DNA.

Perhaps Lou Caverly's essay that questioned, "What is in the payload?" (October 8, 2021) was answered by Dr. Ariyana Love, when she referred to the process of "CRISPR Cast 9 and Blast electro-portation using electrodes on programmable golden nanobots."

"This is how they are targeting the cell organelles of the nuclei. The NIH, Fauci, and DARPA funded this. They're targeting:

1. The neuro cells [prion degeneration], and
2. Embryonic cells [of the vaxxed; due to the vaxxed mother, the offspring's cells are also transfecting.]"

The full horror of the "New Metropolis" stranglehold is evinced by Dr. Love's next statement: "They are gene 'silencing.' *THEY ARE* ***TURNING OFF*** *genes they don't want and programming ones they do want, programming and encoding* ***new genetics.***"

Love concludes: *"THEY'RE WIRING A NEW BRAIN AND NEW NERVOUS SYSTEM, adding a thread to the strands of DNA, so they're taking the 2.0 organic human being and they're transfecting them into a 3.0*

hybrid. *We're under biological attack. The offspring of the mRNA exposed parents are* ***not human.*** *They do not carry God-given genetics. They will be a* ***new species.****"*

Remain God's pure DNA creation. Don't ever subject yourself and your innocent ages 5 to 11 children to this biological scourge—or to any more that arrive with future "plandemics." WE MUST ESCAPE "METROPOLIS" NOW!

—*Elizabeth Cuppett Caverly*

CHAPTER SIXTEEN

A.I., Part Six: "Human Computers"

NaturalNews.com's founder, Mike Adams, had a vital update interview with biotech analyst Karen Kingston, on October 6, 2022. Topics included magnetic hydrogels, tissue engineering, and remote control. A paper in ACS Nano describes how hydrogels can be "scaffolding materials to construct artificial tissues. That ACS article also explains that magnetic nanoparticles can be remotely activated to control cells' behavior that are encapsulated in the hydrogels—if external magnetic fields are applied. The article had this provocative headline—embedded transmission and receiving devices that network to share information, turning human bodies into "cloud" computing platforms. The NaturalNews article went on to say:

> Kingston also reveals how implanted biosynthetic structures have the ability to transmit and receive digitized information, allowing such structures to "network" with each other, even as they reside inside host human bodies. Combined with external AI capabilities that are accelerated by 5G bandwidth speed and low latency, these networking structures can be weaponized against humanity.
>
> One patent cited in this tech is **US11107588B2**, which discusses, "The system comprises a plurality of electronic devices comprising instructions to generate an ID and, when in proximity of another such electronic device, one or both electronic devices transmit/receive the ID to/from the other electronic device."
>
> The technology described in this patent specifically talks about

SARS, MERS, coronavirus, and influenza, or any disease that has "influenza-like symptoms."

—*Elizabeth Cuppett Caverly*

CHAPTER SEVENTEEN

Spectroscopy Findings; The Non-Biological "White Clot"

U.S. embalmer Dr. Richard Hirschman told Dr. Jane Ruby on air in June of 2022 about his bombshell findings—of almost foot-long, branch-like whitish "clots" in people dead after COVID shots. NaturalNews.com, June 12, 2022, posted a stunning article with microscopy photos of strange, seemingly bioengineered, non-human tissue—clot-like structures. These structures, courtesy of Dr. Hirschman, were taken from people who died after getting the COVID shot. Various branch-like appendages resemble what could be genetically bioengineered circuitry. Crystalline areas glow (Luciferase?).

One photo depicts something that looks like a log, covered with tree bark. This "log" has scale-type repetitive markings intermittently along its surface. As part of this biocircuitry interface, there are nanotech wires. People are walking around while mRNA is building these possible embryonic artificial intelligence hook-ups that researchers like Karen Kingston believe one day could be connected to 5G and triggered by it to release a prepared mRNA operating system pathogen that will kill its human carrier.

Happening right now, not in some dark, dystopian A.I. world of the future, your family members and friends are going about their everyday lives, unaware a ticking time bomb is inside their bodies, an escalating assault inside their blood vessels. These are NOT blood clots made of human tissue, as all of us thought.

More information was starting to come out. Corroboration of the veracity of the "white clot" story came from UK funeral director John O'Looney. Here is a partial LifeSiteNews excerpt:

> **UK Funeral Director Tells Steven Crowder About Strange Blood Clots Found In Bodies Of COVID-Vaccinated**
>
> (Kennedy Hall, LifeSiteNews, Thursday, November 3, 2022) The undertaker said that he has spoken to multiple doctors in the British NHS who have confirmed, off the record, that the strange clotting seems to be linked to the mRNA vaccines.
>
> UK-based funeral director John O'Looney appeared on conservative talk-show "Louder with Crowder" to share his experience in finding strange, fibrous blood clots in recently deceased patients who had been "fully vaccinated" against COVID-19. In the interview, O'Looney described the clots as "very much like calamari in their consistency and their elasticity," and said that he has never seen anything like them before.
>
> O'Looney told the podcast's host, Steven Crowder, that his interest in the strange development was piqued when "we had heard a couple of reports of clotting ... when people were coming in who were dying, clearly not from COVID." He said that they found it "very difficult to embalm" to the point where he thought there was an issue with the pump, which he said had never previously happened.
>
> He also told Crowder that he has significant experience in dealing with dead bodies, and that it is his professional duty to "raise any concerns [he has] to the coroner" as per the professional standards of his trade.
>
> O'Looney relayed that he had told the coroner about his concerns and eventually received a response that alleged the clots must have grown after the person had died. "Nothing grows inside your arteries postmortem" he said, "it just doesn't. The only thing that grows in your body postmortem is perhaps mold," he added. "As your body begins to break down, your arteries don't fill up with a white rubbery structure when you die."

O'Looney said that his embalmer likewise expressed that he had never seen anything similar to these clots in his 20 years in the profession.

Later in the interview, Crowder pressed O'Looney on the idea that perhaps these fibrous clots have occurred in both unvaccinated people as well as vaccinated. "It could be the direct result of COVID and the nature of the spike protein, which, of course, we know, we know occurs organically as well," Crowder stated.

O'Looney replied and said that in his experience he has not seen an unvaccinated person with the clots, but said that an embalmer named Richard Hirschman, who like O'Looney has reported the presence of strange clots in deceased people, has only found the same type of clots in one unvaccinated person. However, this unvaccinated person had previously received a blood transfusion sourced from a vaccinated person, according to O'Looney.

O'Looney also said that he has spoken to multiple doctors in the British National Health Service (NHS) who have confirmed, off the record, that the strange clotting seems to be linked to the mRNA vaccines. "Everybody knows," he said.

[A live microscopy of these biostructure clots was conducted by Health Ranger Mike Adams (Alex Jones Show, June 13, 2022). Dr. Jane Ruby and Dr. Richard Hirschman each appeared on a full hour of the program. Mike Adams is speaking in this NaturalNews article excerpt:]

(NaturalNews) EXCLUSIVE: Today we are publishing a series of lab microscopy photos of bizarre clots which are now being routinely found in adults who "suddenly died," usually in a number of months following COVID vaccinations.

These clots are often referred to as "blood clots" but they are nothing at all like normal clots, and they consist of far more than mere blood cells. Unlike normal clots which are gelatinous, almost jelly-like, these so-called "clots" contain extremely large, complex, ***repeating structural elements*** (all shown below) that are clearly being constructed in the blood of the victims who died from these clots.

All of these clots were extracted from patients within a few hours of their death. These are not the result of post-mortem blood stasis. These are *structures* found in blood vessels and arteries. They are not congealed blood.

These structures exhibit the following shocking properties:

- They are tough, fibrous, and resilient, showing material properties similar to small rubber bands.
- They consist of many strands of small, fibrous strands.
- These fibrous strands show repeating patterns of scale-like engineering, as if the body has been programmed to build another life form inside the blood vessels.
- There are strange crystalline-like structures found on these clots, exhibiting transparency and resistance to normal gram staining techniques.
- You will find one example of a structure that appears to resemble a silicon-like biocircuitry or microchip-like structure. We don't yet know what it is.
- One of the photo sets reveals what appears to be a biocircuitry wire which clearly shows repeating patterns and nano-scale interface structures that are assembled in a specific geometry for an unknown purpose.
- When I talk about "biocircuitry or "nanowires," they *resemble* structures that seem to indicate such a purpose, but further research would be needed to confirm these observations.

An embalmer told me that blood emptied from the bodies of these people during embalming often appears to show "chalk-like" white particles which are visible even to the naked eye in certain cases.

What follows here is a stunning look at what appears to be, at first, a micro-scale wire. Zooming it, we see a series of repeating structures along the top that appear to be nano-scale wire interface junctions. The entire "wire" is made of repeating segments, and its outer layer is covered in repeating "scale-like" patterns that actually resemble reptile skin more than anything human. For the record, we don't know what these structures are. However, it's clear this doesn't belong anywhere in the circulatory system. Finally, this fiber is not simply a human hair. It is firmly attached to the blood clot and when I tried to remove it, it would not tear away easily. This is not a contamination issue; it is a structure emanating from the clot itself. Everything you see here came out of a human being's blood vessels:

What is all this?

We don't yet know what all these structures are. We know what they are not, however: They are not simply clotted blood cells. If they were, then at the 1500x magnification shown in the last photo, above, we would be able to see individual blood cells. These are not blood cells, **they are protein structures.** Protein structures circulating in the blood like this, building up over time, are clearly being constructed by the body's cells. The ribosomes in the cells instruct the body what proteins to construct. These ribosomes are hijacked by mRNA gene therapy injections, which overwrite new instructions to the cells, causing them to manufacture something other than human.

I believe the structures you are seeing above are the result of mRNA protein synthesis instructions which have been injected into people under the false umbrella of "vaccines." **Only independent scientists, labs, and journalists will dare tell the truth about these clots.** In conclusion, they are not "blood" clots. They are structures in the blood. They are "structural clots" or "fibrous clots" that are extremely large and are being constructed inside the body over time.

My grave concern is that every person who has been injected with mRNA instructions may be constructing these fibrous structures inside their bodies at this very minute, and that it's only a matter of time before they block major arteries or cause heart attacks, strokes or other acute causes of "Sudden Adult Death Syndrome" (SADS). I believe these structures may very well explain why so many seemingly healthy adults are suddenly dying.

[In this excerpt below, Mike discusses the results of his ICP-MS elemental analysis:]

EXCLUSIVE: NaturalNews releases post-vaccine clot ICP-MS elemental analysis results, comparing clots to human blood ... findings reveal these clots are NOT "blood" clots

(Mike Adams, NaturalNews, Wednesday, August 17, 2022)

We are now releasing ICP-MS lab test results that compare the elemental composition of human blood to the elemental composition of a clot sample taken from the body of a person who received a COVID vaccination and then subsequently died.

[Interestingly, Lou Caverly's speculation on us being turned into the Tin Man, along with Karen Kingston's "trackable, traceable A.I." (with possible 5G activating vaccine nanotech operating systems) may all be ***reality***. Mike Adam's next charts suggest this. ***Conductivity is the "power" word of the hour***.]

ICP-MS analysis results reveal that these clots are not made of blood—they are not "blood clots." They are not simply made of congealed blood. How do we know this? Because the elemental ratios and densities are vastly different. Consider the following comparison chart. Notice the stark differences between the elemental concentrations in blood vs. clot among nutritive "marker" elements such as iron and magnesium:

Element	Blood Results	Clot Results
Mg (magnesium)	35 ppm	1.7 ppm
K (potassium)	1893 ppm	12.5 ppm
Fe (iron)	462 ppm	20.6 ppm
Zn (zinc)	7.9 ppm	2.4 ppm

Cl (chlorine)	930,000 ppm	290,000 ppm
P (phosphorous)	1130 ppm	4900 ppm

As you can see, the post-vaccine clot sample **only contains 4.4% of the iron that would be seen in human blood.** This alone is confirmation that this clot is not a "blood clot." In addition, note the near-total lack of potassium (K) in the clot sample. The clot contains less than 0.6% of the potassium as human blood. It's a similar story with magnesium, too.

Several electrically conductive elements were higher in the clot.

In addition to the nutritive elements shown above, we noticed a peculiar pattern among electrically conductive elements such as sodium (Na), aluminum (Al) and tin (Sn). For the following table, please note that the tin and sodium results come from a separate "semiquant" report which is less accurate than the "fullquant" analysis used for all the other elements shown here. In essence, the semiquant numbers are accurate in terms of relative concentrations from one sample to the next, but they are not compared to calibrated external samples, so the actual (absolute) concentration reported does not have the confidence interval of the fullquant results:

Element	**Blood Results**	**Clot Results**
Na (sodium)	1050 ppm*	1500 ppm*
Sn (tin)	163 ppb*	942 ppb*
Al (aluminum)	1.3 ppm	1.6 ppm

* = SemiQuant results, not FullQuant

With sodium being nearly 50% higher in the clot, and tin showing an increase of 588%, we can only conclude that **the self-assembling clot is, in effect, "harvesting" or concentrating certain elements from**

> **circulating blood as clot assembly is taking place.** It is noteworthy that many of these elements are conductive. Aluminum, for example, is the most common alternative to copper for use in electrical wiring. Sodium is an alkali metal that is highly conductive, and tin is used as the primary component in solder alloys used to manufacture or repair circuit boards.
>
> One conclusion is inescapable: **The clot is almost entirely lacking key marker elements that would be present in human blood (such as iron and potassium) yet shows significantly higher concentrations of elements that are used in electronics and circuitry.**
>
> My own professional opinion is that these clots are not living structures. They appear to be self-assembling dead biostructures, from what we can see so far. Prions, for example, are self-assembling but non-living biostructures too. They are essentially mis-folded proteins that spread throughout the brain (or other regions), causing morphological alterations that nullify both the normal structure and function of neurological cells. Something does not have to be alive in order to be self-assembling. Even viruses, as described by traditional virology, are dead structures which are nevertheless self-assembling and can "grow" in size and mass in terms of their aggregate population.

These were stunning articles from Mike Adams with microscopy photos of strange, seemingly bioengineered, non-human tissue, clot-like structures. The bizarre structures, courtesy of Dr. Hirschman, were taken from people who died after getting the COVID shot. Various branch-like appendages resemble what could be genetically bioengineered circuitry. Crystalline areas glow (Luciferase?).

One photo depicts something that looks like a log, covered with tree bark. This "log" has scale-type repetitive markings intermittently along its surface. As part of this bio-circuitry interface, there are nanotech wires.

People are walking around while mRNA is building these possible embryonic artificial intelligence hook-ups that researchers like Karen Kingston believe one day could be connected to 5G and triggered by it to release a prepared mRNA operating system pathogen that will kill its human carrier. Happening right now, not in some dark, dystopian A.I. world of the future, where your family members and friends are going about their everyday lives, unaware. A ticking time bomb is inside their bodies, an escalating assault inside their blood vessels. These are NOT blood clots made of human tissue.

Some signs that these artificial mRNA constructs are dangerously cutting off circulation in the body are blackened, necrotic fingers and toes (now dubbed "COVID toes or fingers"). When the process worsens, circulation is seriously stifled in the heart or brain, and "unexpected death" may occur.

This death by "diabolical stealth" is how the globalist depopulationists will slaughter billions, unseen, undetected. Stalin and Mao were involved in child's play compared to these present Big Pharma fiends.

Some Chapter Seventeen concluding thoughts:

In August 2023, we must note that widespread cowardice of any other labs remained, in that no other brave labs stepped up to duplicate Mike Adams's spectroscopy analysis. The mainstream press, too, continued to distort the truth, one of these lies being a variation of another long-standing deception.

Barbara Loe Fisher and other leading medical experts who expose harm done by childhood vaccines have discussed for decades the so-called "Sudden Infant Death Syndrome." They have revealed that a number of innocent parents have been arraigned on false charges that they shook the baby in question before its demise. Despite the very strong evidence for vaccine links, this Death by Big Pharma has escaped notice.

It is just amazing that this old lie has been expanded to help cover up COVID vaccine death links. Yes, after Operation Warp Speed, we suddenly began hearing all over the news about "Sudden Adult Death Syndrome." This is a silly scenario of unbelievability to distract the populace from their awakening horror as they actually begin to question why so many young, top world athletes have dropped dead shortly after COVID shots.

At this time, what is the state of God's church house. God is a jealous God. None—not even famed and powerful church leaders—will prosper and live in peace if they continue to lie and promote the globalists' plan—a hidden "Green Genocide," planning to starve billions as they thwart CO2, so necessary for plants and animals.

This, of course, accompanies the final fruition of the COVID Casualty Agenda that obscenely reaches its Murder, Inc. peak when they approved homicidal COVID clot shots for tiny babies in their cribs. It was not enough for the children aged 5 to 11 to have been injured in large numbers by these mRNA "vaccines."

We wonder what top church leaders will say about this August 4, 2023, AP headline, "Babies should get recently approved drug for RSV, CDC says." Probably nothing. Top church leaders in America said nary a word much earlier when the U.S. College of Obstetricians actually recommended that pregnant women get COVID shots. **That silence was followed by a huge number of tragic miscarriages**. Now, we look again at the latest August 2023 headline, "Babies should get recently approved drug for RSV, CDC says." This will be a one-time shot for infants born before or during the RSV [respiratory syncytial virus] season and for those less than 8 months old before the season starts. This drug, Beyfortus, the AP says, is expected to cost $495 per dose.

We recently heard from a radio listener that her church pastor was quite interested in knowing more about the satanic New World Order plan. So, we recommended the listener present the pastor with what we both consider to be the best Christian documentary film of the year, "Klaus Schwab, The Third Reich, and the COVID-19 Holocaust" (available at swrc.com). Every video segment is unforgettable in its uncompromised truth-telling. Sadly, the latest news from the listener is, "The man at the chapel who is in charge of okaying the DVDs to be put in the church library refused permission." The church representative actually remarked, "they are *not for* ***this church***!"

Who will you serve in the years ahead, even as judgment from God likely sends America into further lawlessness, chaos, and perhaps even captivity? ... A great separation is starting ... The United Methodist

Churches in Georgia have split off … Will you take a stand for God's righteousness? … Will you tell the hard truths and witness to others about salvation in Jesus?

"As for me and my house, we will serve the Lord" —Joshua 24:15

—*Elizabeth Cuppett Caverly*

CHAPTER EIGHTEEN

The Strange Serpentine Scenario

THE SNAKE VENOM PEPTIDES ARE NOT GOING AWAY

These are some essential facts from Dr. Ardis' October 25 and 28 interviews with Stew Peters and Dr. Jane Ruby:

» More than 36 different venoms (20 from snakes and others from snails) were incorporated in the COVID bioweapon.
» Deadly "Crown of Thorns" starfish venom was used. [Note the "Crucifixion of Christ" symbol in this satanic venom plan.]
» A total of 15 different conotoxins (snail venoms) were found in COVID patients' blood in a vital study done by Italian researchers. Why has this study been ignored by the world? Did Biden's COVID-19 Community Corps (against COVID "disinformation") suppress it?
» Two Chinese snakes, the krait and king cobra were used ... Interestingly, Dr. Jane Ruby commented, "Why were 800,000 Chinese students studying in America exempt from taking the COVID inoculations?"
» A patent from 1999 for synthetic conotoxin peptides is co-owned by these two institutions:
  1. The Salk Institute. Recall the polio vaccine and the "quiet" later cancer deaths of perhaps thousands caused by SV-40, the contaminant Simian (monkey) virus.
  2. The University of Utah. In addition, Ardis reveals that NIH (The National Institutes of Health) awarded grants that led to these institutions obtaining these patents.

» In addition, Ardis informs us that Clemson University Children's Hospital owns some conotoxin patents! Doesn't this equate to Georgetown University advocating "trans" mutilation surgery on children in their training program for physicians? This is "Molech Body and Soul Murder of Children, Inc." More than a heavy millstone, according to the Bible, will be placed around the necks of these sinister planners and participants in harming God's beloved little ones.

» According to Ardis' findings, polysorbate 80 and polyethylene glycol are found in the COVID shots, and the polysorbate 80 "punches holes in the blood/brain barrier (thus facilitating neurological damage as the venom intrudes into the brain.)" It is the injury to the cranial nerves that causes COVID patients to lose their sense of taste and smell. If polysorbate 80 is in flu shots, Ardis says, it could also allow aluminum into the brain.

» Ardis says, "Every single side effect, including the onset of myocarditis, can be attributed to venom." Since the 1800s, myocarditis has been documented to be one of the side effects of snake venom exposure.

» Stew Peters responds, "There's nothing to say multiple things can't be part of the shots." [We add that it is true, too, in the case of the original pandemic COVID bioweapon.]

» Ardis: "It looks like they weaponized snake venom." There is research on nanoparticle hydrogels that indicates these (1) self-replicate and (2) cause blood clotting.

» "What about the people who 'died suddenly'?" Stew wonders. [*Died Suddenly* is also the name of the new movie releasing at Stew Peters in early November.] Stew says, "Many of these people reach out, spinning around before they drop dead." Dr. Ardis responds, "There is a visual hallucination from the snake venom when it crosses the blood/brain barrier. Research shows that after snake bites, people can have schizophrenic delusions."

» An NIH website, "Serum Sickness," actually reports a day 13 window when myocarditis results from venom.

- » Ardis tells Stew that venom peptides are circulating in the body as a person's DNA is making the peptides [Via mRNA operating systems].
- » When Peters and Ardis asked Dr. Robert Malone (self-alleged creator of mRNA technology) about "venom," they "got no answer."
- » Utah State University has done genetic engineering with E. coli, along with toxins. This, Ardis says, is to make the body more able to produce venom. This apparent facilitation of venom production has also been linked to yeast over-production in humans. For this reason, Dr. Ardis says, physicians should be aware that, in diabetic patients, COVID disease escalation into a more serious form may have yeast or E. coli playing a role that should be understood in patient treatment protocols.
- » Dr. Ardis: "Phospholipid A-2 is the enzyme responsible for killing the COVID-19 patients. Another enzyme, SPLA-2 shreds tissue of body organs as it fights a virus." SPLAC was first found in cobras!
- » Some remedies, Ardis suggests, may be somewhat helpful in mitigating venom effects. These, according to him, include: bromelain, aloe vera, vitamin C, EDTA, and resveratrol.

Mike Adams, Health Ranger (NaturalNews.com, April 15, 2021) gave facts about "Pharma Snakes":

- » Reptile venoms can be weaponized and made into biological weapons. Protein sequences are provided by the venom library companies, allowing gain-of-function research to engineer venom peptides into viral payloads or mRNA therapeutics. Because venoms are poisons, the knowledge of how to engineer and synthesize those poisons at the amino acid level is also knowledge of how to build biological or chemical weapons.
- » Dozens of pharmaceuticals derived entirely from animal venom already exist. Many are FDA approved.
- » Pharma appears to be HIDING the venom origins of their

products, making few or no disclosures on marketing websites about the actual origin of their drugs.

- Nearly zero doctors or patients know about the venom origins of venom-derived medications.
- Venom molecules and venom peptides are mass synthesized in pharmaceutical factories. This is a common practice. This is referred to by numerous scientific and bioscience resources, including the World Economic Forum.
- Because venom peptides are stable in solution, they can be weaponized and mass-produced, then distributed via air, water, food, or contact surfaces. This means that it is *entirely plausible* that mass poisoning via venom peptides could be accomplished through the water supply, the food supply, or dropped on cities via drones, etc.
- Some toxins are skin-penetrating and can be absorbed merely by TOUCH (not a venom, but a toxin or poison). This was all admitted in an Ecohealth Alliance proposal to DARPA, as covered in this story: "Leaked DARPA document, DRASTIC analysis confirms attack on humanity using aerosolized, skin-penetrating nanoparticle spike proteins."
- Venoms and venom peptides produced for pharma are so stable that they survive stomach acid, which means the venom peptides are stable in solution, including in rather acidic (reactive) solutions. This means they do not automatically break down in city water, either. If venom toxins were not highly stable molecules, they would not be very good venoms in the first place. As ToxinTech explains, "millions of years of evolution" have perfected the functionality of these molecules.

Mike Adams has this bombshell update at NaturalNews.com, Friday, November 4, 2022:

"Venom theory" proven correct as scientists confirm presence of dozens of venom peptides in COVID-19 victims

A study published in the F1000 Research journal, indexed by PubMed

Central and available on the National Library of Medicine website (https://www.ncbi.nlm.nih.gov/pmc/articles/PMC8772524/) is titled, "Toxin-like peptides in plasma, urine and fecal samples from COVID-19 patients."

This study used HPLC (liquid chromatography) combined with mass spec instruments to identify the presence of dozens of venom peptide components in the feces and blood plasma of COVID-19 victims. Authored by Carlo Brogna and other Italian researchers, the study, "reports the identification of toxin-like peptides in COVID-19 patients by application of the Liquid Chromatography Surface-Activated Chemical Ionization—Cloud Ion Mobility Mass Spectrometry."

The full list of toxic peptides and venom peptide components identified in the bodies of COVID-19 victims include:

Conotoxin Pu6.1	Conotoxin Vi15a
Putative alpha-conotoxin Qc alphaL-1	Conotoxin 10
Rho-conotoxin TIA	Kunitz-type serine protease inhibitor
conotoxin Cal9.1a	Alpha-conotoxin Pu1.5
Conotoxin Fla16d	Phospholipase A2 MALT0035C
Phospholipase A2 AP-PLA2-I	Acidic phospholipase A2 PePLA2
Basic phospholipase A2 BFPA	Basic phospholipase A2 PL-X
Complement factor B Ba fragment	Acidic phospholipase A2 homolog textilotoxin D chain
Acidic phospholipase A2 homolog textilotoxin D chain	Venom prothrombin activator pseutarin-C non-catalytic subunit

Coagulation factor V	Venom prothrombin activator oscutarin-C non-catalytic subunit
Short neurotoxin 4	Conotoxin Cl9.6
Zinc metalloproteinase-disintegrin-like halysase	Alpha-elapitoxin-Oh2b
Sigma-conotoxin GVIIIA	Conotoxin Mr15.2
Conotoxin mr3g	Contryphan-R
Snake venom metalloprotease inhibitor 02D01	Bradykinin-potentiating and C-type natriuretic peptides
Bradykinin-potentiating and C-type natriuretic peptides	Zinc metalloproteinase/ disintegrin

—*Elizabeth Cuppett Caverly*

CHAPTER NINETEEN

Six Months Later—Update on Serpentine Scenario

October 13, 2022

» April 18—Stew Peters reports over 6 million people have watched the Dr. Brian Ardis documentary, *Watch the Water*, that provided strong medical journal documentation that inclusion of cobra-venom peptides occurred in the COVID "vaccines."

» April 18—Dr. Jane Ruby hears from a researcher who claims to have identified king cobra venom in the contents of a Pfizer COVID-19 vaccine vial: "snake venom organoids."

» April 19—Indomitable COVID investigator Karen Kingston gives Stew Peters a report from her latest digging into incriminating patents. She reports:

A. The full sequence of the COVID "virus" can be seen to include elements from bats, mice, the Middle Eastern virus, and more. [We recall our essay that included Dr. Judy Mikovits's description of COVID that mentioned such things as leukemia virus from mice.]

2. Two key figures appear to have been NIAID's Barney Graham and Moderna's Jason McClellan. According to Kingston, they filed the spike-protein patent in April 2019!! Amazing! How did they file this even before they had access to the sequence?

3. According to Kingston, there is evidence that Graham and McClellan added the snake venom to the spike protein.

4. In 2017, why did the NIH file a vaccine patent that in Section

9 states, "The vaccine in some embodiment can deliver a molecule of chemical weapon of biowarfare or a toxin."

It seems an extensive network is in place involving these heretofore unknown Ardis cobra aspects of COVID. Kingston continues:

E. Eco Health Alliance's involvement working on 180 sequences
F. The University of Pittsburgh [Recall the 10 gunshots that silenced University of Pittsburgh researcher Bing Lieu, who was about to announce findings on COVID] took 38 European COVID patients, and scientists looked for the protein causing the "multi-inflammatory systems." These researchers looked for toxins. The PRA was published in *The Lancet.* They found the krait, cobra venom, and rabies virus, plus the HIV glycoprotein 120 [The "Gain of Function"?]
G. Karen Kingston states she has the patent for the spike protein and that it is a separate patent from the mRNA.
H. In addition, the master patent for mRNA, the World Patent for Moderna, #0402, interestingly states it "can deliver a toxin." Kingston adds, "The patents say the vaccine is a bioweapon."
I. Kingston recounts the strange reaction of Dr. Robert Malone on the "Joe Rogan Show." (Dr. Malone claims to be the inventor of mRNA, though other credible reports list two University of Pennsylvania researchers as having developed the mRNA process.) When Joe Rogan asked Malone about "gene editing," Dr. Malone laughed ominously and said there were brown monkeys that had HIV and "Let's put that into the mRNA technology." In a later interview with Stew Peters, Dr. Robert Malone said he knows much more that he cannot tell for fear of losing his medical license. Stew Peters stated that he himself had had his home surrounded twice by a SWAT team, then caustically remarked on the many media figures and politicians too cowardly to bring out the horrific truth about COVID. Later, going even into 2023, a shocking lawsuit

brought against valiant Dr. Jane Ruby by Dr. Robert Malone was still pending. Was this a frivolous legal action to "shut up" an uncompromising truth-teller? The serpent COVID story moves on.

» Dr. Ben Marvel (who has treated 15,000 COVID patients) calls for more testing, for Italian studies show the venom peptides *were* in COVID patients. Marvel's opinion is that perhaps the venom peptides were not the "main poison" of the COVID shots. He remarked, *"FIVE BILLION people have had the shots."* In Ardis' Brighteon.com interviews, he presented evidence suggesting the drug REMDESIVIR CONTAINS FREEZE-DRIED COBRA VENOM. Marvel responds: "We need to test Remdesivir to see if the venoms are there. If so, ban it!" Marvel comments further, *"Over half the world's population has been poisoned by the COVID shots. DR. LUC MONTAGNIER SAID HALF OF THOSE WILL DIE."*

» April 20—Dr. Jane Ruby reports that 50 percent of the contents of the COVID-19 vaccine vials can be "undeclared." So this means, she explains, that at any given time, these COVID shots can have different materials even within the same lot number!

» April 20—Sara Sugden, mother of an autistic son and vaccine researcher, reports that CHILDREN HAVE LARGE, ROBUST THYMUS ORGANS, whereas elderly persons have thymuses that are weak and shrunken and can no longer produce new T-cells. This may be the explanation for why children were largely unaffected by COVID. Their thymuses could recognize "brand new" pathogens when the older people's couldn't.

» April 20—Sugden also comments on the cobra-COVID connection: ***"The venom affects your cells in a specific way that allows the graphene oxide to communicate with 5G, so all of your cells have voltage-gated ion channels."*** Elements like calcium and sodium are involved, too. The 5G keeps the membrane open and the graphene oxide "cooks on your skin." On the skin is where researchers found spike proteins accumulating. The use of 5G shows the calcium and sodium at high levels. **And the graphene**

will be used in the process to help identify you, biometrically.

- April 22—Dr. Jane Ruby reports that Dr. Brian Ardis and Dr. Zandré Botha, expert blood microscopy expert, met with her to discuss the little round ***"bubbly circles"*** that have been seen in COVID vaccine vial contents over the last 6 to 8 months. *Matching up with the research findings of the Herschek Institute (their work on **extracting snake venom and making little organoids,** synthetic venom peptides), **these newest particles,** lately observed in the vials, **appear to be the same phenomenon.*** Dr. Jane says, ***"These cells are still live!"*** She wonders whether the Red Cross is "paid off" —still no program of blood donor surveillance for spike proteins ...
- Late April—An alternative health proponent suggests that using zinc and melatonin may be of benefit to treat stubborn "long COVID" cases. If the cobra venom is part of the cause, these are known to help fight the effects of the venom. ***Is snake venom the cause of the damage to the cranial nerves and the loss of taste and smell in COVID patients?***
- Early Fall Update 2022—Karen Kingston reiterates on the "Stew Peters Show" that she has located the patents for king and krait cobra venom as used by the sinister vaccine lab "enthusiasts."

—*Elizabeth Cuppett Caverly*

CHAPTER 20

Death by Eugenics: Then and Now

(Divided Kingdom Radio, November 28, 2021)

In the 1930s the elites in many states had bought into the pseudoscience of eugenics—the belief that the American people (as well as other nationalities) could be "bred" to produce an improved species. Earlier proponents, like Francis Galton in England, thought that the "best" individuals should marry to have superior offspring. But, in the United States, the concept had been strongly influenced by Social Darwinism—only the strong would survive. Hence, the weak would have to be eliminated.

As a consequence, many states instituted compulsory sterilization laws. Author Edwin Black states that almost half of the victims were in California. In Virginia, poor whites in rural areas, blacks, epileptics, and others were picked up by law enforcement and taken to state hospitals where they were sterilized, often without their knowledge. Most of them were ordinary people who happened to have been born into poverty. Some were told only years later why they could have no children. Others were never told at all. They were classified as "feeble-minded," although just what that meant was not explained. At least 60,000 people were sterilized across America before the practice was ended.

A half century later, one victim, who was ashamed to use his real name, went by the pseudonym "Buck Smith." He told a newspaper reporter, "Eventually you knew your time would come. ... We weren't growed up enough to think about it. We didn't know what it meant" [Edwin Black, *War Against the Weak*, p. 5].

The American eugenics movement strongly influenced the plans of Adolf Hitler when he came to power. "Hitler and his race hygienists carefully crafted eugenic legislation modeled on laws already introduced across America. ... Hitler himself regularly communicated with American eugenicists from New York to California" [Black, p. 277]. There is a direct link between the sterilizations in the United States and the Holocaust in Nazi Germany.

Once again, turn the clock face forward to 2021. Have things really changed? We hear reports of Australian indigenous citizens being kidnapped by military troops and taken to quarantine camps. There are even Australian reports of victims being thrown down and inoculated by force. This is in violation of the first Nuremberg Code, written in the aftermath of World War II. To prevent future atrocities like the ones committed by the Nazi doctors, the first of these codes reads: "The voluntary consent of the human subject is absolutely essential."

And what about the United States? As mentioned previously, Dr. Jane Ruby reported on November 22, 2021, that the mass vaccination clinic run by James Kyle Turnbo was luring young children to get COVID vaccinations, accompanied by Santa, lollipops, and other fun enticements. Turnbo is "double dipping" into his federal loan to make more money.

"BIOWEAPONS FOR BABIES" could also be the slogan for the child COVID mRNA gene shots being administered at East Tennessee Mercy Hospital. But Dr. David Berry and the Blacksburg, Virginia, Pediatric Clinic got a head start on all the others, hastening to begin the dangerous new child vax experiments around the first week of November. [Note: the setting of rural Tennessee and Virginia is very reminiscent of the locations of the 1930s secret sterilizations.]

Dr. David Berry, of Blacksburg Pediatric Center (owned by the Privia Group, which is almost 100 percent controlled by Goldman Sachs) gives out popsicles and stickers to unsuspecting children. Dr. Berry states proudly, "We've seen a huge response and are ***humbled by it! ...***"

Vaccination mandates are trying to take hold here in America. Can we really call the vaccinations "voluntary" when failure to take the jab will result in loss of livelihood? Remember, Hitler's early laws deprived

Jews and certain others of the means to practice a profession. The death camps and Final Solution were on the horizon. Where is the outrage at sending our tiniest children into the fires of Molech, ***even as the infamous Dr. Fauci calls for injecting infants next?***

—Lou Caverley

CHAPTER 21

Bombshell Leak: COVID Vax Companies Use Nazi Code Lot Numbers to Track Deaths

January 6, 2022

The so-called "omicron" COVID variant (letters rearrange to spell "moronic") is surging in the U.S. and all over the world. The obituaries in the newspapers here on the Eastern Shore of Maryland continue to show an unusually high ratio of deaths in which people "pass away peacefully or unexpectedly at home." Many are African-American men in their fifties and sixties. One 29-year-old man who unexpectedly left Earth was photographed in his coffin. Scott Davison, CEO of Indiana's One America Life Insurance Company reports that for the third quarter of 2021 working-age deaths (18–64) were up 40 percent over pre-pandemic numbers of 2020. This is about 3,000 extra American deaths in one day! And about 90,000 extra American deaths in a month! Health Ranger Mike Adams (Brighteon.com) predicts one million excess deaths in 2022 compared to 2019.

Dr. Jane Ruby before Christmas valiantly ferreted out the truth of post-vaccine COVID clot-shots: airline pilots' deaths, military men's and women's injuries, and now she highlights the barbaric inoculations of 5- to 11-year-olds. People can no longer ignore tragedies like the unspeakable case of the 8-year-old Wyoming boy who post-jab went into a coma, had a heart attack, and is now left with myocarditis. Perhaps under the spell God mentions in Isaiah 29:10–15, the Wyoming boy's mother posts on her social media site pictures of her wan-looking son eating his first meal after coming out of the coma. She murmurs enthusiastically, "I'm so glad he got vaccinated. There are so many sick people around."

Dr. Reiner Fuellmich has alluded to the possibility of marked differences in vials of COVID vaccines. Some other researchers postulated there were differing vial contents being designated for various geographical areas, perhaps targeting different population types. Now, today, January 6, Dr. Jane Ruby reports to Stew Peters (Brighteon.com) this huge breaking story. Purposeful "truth hackers" went into Pfizer, Moderna, and Johnson and Johnson (Janssen) internet systems. What these researchers found is right in line with the German Nazi obsession with order—evil classifications and operations like the methodical IBM punch cards, functional yellow stars forced universally on 1940s European Jewry, and finally, the super-efficient Zyklon B "shower" killings and crematoria to erase the whole record of murderous activity.

Dr. Jane Ruby gives the findings of these latest courageous hackers. Apparently, COVID 19 vaccines are an experimental "lethal dose" test—intentionally designed to export *illness and injury* to the E.U. but to *cause* death in the U.S.A. [We have to ask ourselves, could some of this purpose be to rid the U.S. of more Second Amendment gun-carrying men from ages 18 to 64, as well as specifically to cut down on defense readiness numbers of U.S. military and states' National Guard members?]

Dr. Ruby reports the COVID drug producers actually list lot numbers in categories of tainted batches so they can track their death and illness "success"! Some categories are as follows: Pfizer's most dangerous vials for children are coded as "EW," the deadliest lot of all being "EW0182." Its second deadliest for children begins with "FA" or "FC." For adults, Pfizer's most harmful is coded as "EN"; second deadliest for adults is "ER." Moderna's most dangerous lots for all ages end in "20A." "Super-toxic" vials are coded "J," "K," "L," or "M' in the middle of the number [go to "Most Dangerous Lots"—HowBad.info]. One member on the analysis team for the hacking results was Dr. Michael Yeadon, the well-known former Pfizer high-level employee whistleblower.

Ruby says the "EW" lot is responsible for almost all adverse events in children: all ER visits, all hospitalizations, all life-threatening events, disabilities, and deaths. All these lots are in circulation, and there can be as many as 1.5 million doses in a lot. Dr. Ruby points out that experimental "lethal dose" testing has always been done with animals only, never people. COVID shots' "lethal dose" testing is being administered worldwide to human beings, certainly without "informed consent." This covert subjugation is against all ethical and regulatory rules. The companies are actually embedding codes within lot numbers so they can monitor which are toxic, which cause disabilities, and what type of disabilities. For example, Moderna lot 011L20A; the 20A, again, is the deadliest code. (These designations were running from mid-November 2021 to at least December 16, 2021.)

In December, truth about COVID vaccines was being stonewalled everywhere. The mainstream media suppressed any mention of Robert F. Kennedy, Jr.'s book, *The Real Anthony Fauci*, even as it became the best-selling book in America. A population "killing machine" appears to have had diabolical Nazi-like success.

God is indeed greater than all the horrors of evil we face this January 2022. It is understandable for us, even as Christians, to have times of grieving those lost and mourning for our pre-"plandemic" lives. But remember the case of Pastor Dr. Richard Wurmbrand, imprisoned for thirteen years underground in Romania. (He went blind in those years from being held in darkness). In 1972 or '73, I actually saw him in person. He was a visiting speaker at a small Baptist church in Lanham, Maryland. Still quite fragile, he sat on a chair, sometimes encouraged by his wife nearby. Yet when one sees his photo on a book jacket about a decade later, Wurmbrand again looks triumphantly vigorous and healthy. He had emerged victorious, writing books about his life story to encourage and lift God's people. God, indeed did a miracle in this great pastor's restoration.

Jesus Christ can renew and refresh us, too, even in our present national nightmare if we choose to be truly His. A great separation has begun. The wheat is being divided from the chaff.

For Christians, there is no compromise. Your choice is to inoculate yourself with aborted fetal cell vaccines, or to keep God's DNA He created in your body, pure—as you put your complete hope and trust in Jesus Christ, Savior of the World.

—*Elizabeth Cuppett Caverly*

CHAPTER TWENTY-TWO

Gestapo, COVID Quarantine Camps, Medical Police State, U.S. Trains Australia

[Moving chronologically through the year 2021, we track the connection between despotism in both America and Australia. May 20, 2021, had this report on the odious new U.S.A. Stormtroopers. There were some early COVID vaccine death statistics:]

> (Great Game India, Journal on Geopolitics & International Relations, May 20, 2021)
>
> In Dallas County, uniformed US military troops went around vaccinating Americans in bars and restaurants. Dallas County Health and Human Services organized a pop-up COVID-19 vaccine drive with uniformed US Army National Guard soldiers going around bars and restaurants with vaccines.
>
> They were spotted walking around Deep Ellum randomly trying to vaccinate people and bar goers who haven't been vaccinated yet in Dallas.

[It is truly unconscionable to force a bioweapon injection on human beings whose reason is impaired by alcohol. Once more, we have in this gestapo military exercise exactly what Edwin Black wrote about in *The War Against the Weak.*]

In this time of COVID and coming chaos, many people don't know that the mindset of Hitler's eugenics T-4 Plan to euthanize handicapped Germans originated not in Germany, but here in the United States. The book we mentioned, Edwin Black's *The War Against the Weak,* details awful eugenics activities in 1920s and '30s America. Planned Parenthood founder Margaret Sanger made sure her close friend, Ernst Rudin in Germany, was informed and recruited into this dark ideal to restrict and/or kill "useless eaters."

So, here in 2021, it was very interesting to see the U.S. apparently in the forefront, taking the lead to institute a medical police state. Later in the year, the country of Australia would copy those tactics. Indeed later in 2023, there comes forth strong documentation that the "American Babylon" government was "the head of the snake."

QUARANTINE CAMPS

World Net Daily

Shock executive order greenlights quarantines, involuntary commitment amid COVID fears

'The pieces add up to a very scary picture! People need to wake up'

An executive order signed quietly by Tennessee's Republican governor greenlights the National Guard and State Guard to implement quarantines and involuntary commitment of citizens "in connection with certain health care and emergency services operations," with the governor specifically concerned about "an increase in COVID-19 cases."

Gov. Bill Lee signed Executive Order 83 on Friday "with little fanfare" according to Tennessee Stands, an influential conservative coalition.

The group says it found some of the provisions in the executive order "exceptionally concerning," including:

» "Discretion to utilize National Guard and State Guard members in connection with certain health care and emergency services operations."

» "Telephone assessments for involuntary commitment cases are permitted."

» "Temporary quarantine and isolation facilities may be constructed."

AUSTRALIA— QUEENSLAND COMMENCES IN-HOME QUARANTINE

Australian state launches new check-in system to track quarantined residents, those who fail to respond get a visit from cops

(Arsenio Toleda, Natural News, Friday, September 17, 2021) The government of Australia's northeastern state of Queensland has launched a new check-in system for its residents' in-home quarantine, requiring them to answer a randomly-timed text message within 10 minutes. If they do not, *police officers will show up at their doorsteps.* The new rules went into effect immediately after they were crafted. They were pushed by the state government of the ruling left-wing Labor Party after health authorities discovered just one new locally transmitted COVID-19 case. The message will feature a link that the recipient has to open and respond to within 10 minutes.

Additionally, *Queensland Health's* new rules require residents in-home quarantine to keep their mobile data and geolocation services on their mobile phones activated at all times. This means even if residents respond within 10 minutes, they might still get a compliance visit from the *Queensland Police Service* if their response was outside an "acceptable geolocation range."

"This means *Queensland Health* will be able to ensure individuals in-home quarantine are at the residence they're lawfully required to be at," said D'Ath. "It specifically allows authorities to identify if anybody is away from their approved residence." The new restrictions will apply to all close contacts of confirmed COVID-19 cases. Potential breaches in the restrictions will be assessed by the QPS to identify whether further action is required. D'Ath justified the system by saying it would "enable real-time *monitoring of compliance.*" "For more than 18 months, text messages, phone calls, and random inspections for compliance have long been the hallmarks of our home quarantine system, but as the virus evolves, so must our response," said D'Ath.

Any Queensland resident who violates their home quarantine can be fined up to AU$13,785 ($10,082), spend up to six months in jail, and be forced out of their homes and told to go to state-recognized quarantine hotels. They must pay for their mandated stays at the hotels. (Related: MEDICAL POLICE STATE: Elderly Australian couple forced to drive three hundred miles to quarantine hotel after filling out form incorrectly.)

The city of Lismore in New South Wales, which is less than a hundred miles to the south of the Queensland capital of Brisbane, has around 40,000 residents and has been placed under lockdown due to the one positive case.

KAREN KINGSTON LETS THE SECRETS OUT: G2G APP WORLD BONDAGE PLAN

(Elizabeth C. Caverly, Divided Kingdom Radio Monologue, October 19, 2021)

October 12, 2021, on Brighteon.com, whistleblower Karen Kingston exposed tyranny of the Australian COVID quarantine app G2G. Also revealed was the sinister plan for worldwide Artificial Intelligence (A.I.) of the Organization for Economic Cooperation and Development. The U.S. has made a commitment to this group. Part of a key associated publication is section 0060, "Prioritized Strategies for Pandemic Influenza Vaccine" for 27 Countries of the E.U. and Global Health Security Action Group (now 38 countries).

Kingston found that the "operating mRNA system" with its strange colors and seemingly "self-aware" entities analyzed lately by Drs. Carrie Madej and Zandré Botha is, in truth, "an obedience tool." This "obedience platform," she says, if not stopped, will become an "execution platform."

Patent 2021/0082583, section 0378, states one may need to download an app that helps the government with COVID quarantine procedures. The app, "G2G Now," is presently functioning in Australia.

G2G Now:

» Users receive a "push" notification to check-in.
» They have a five-minute window to take a "selfie" and send it to the app.
» "G2G Now" then matches the image and location with the person's registered details.
» This is to ensure compliance with the user's quarantine directions.
» If the "target" does not respond ("Sleeping?" "Showering?") within the five-minute window, a second "check-in" request follows shortly.
» If the G2G-targeted person misses the second request, the app prompts the person to give a reason.
» Police will then determine what ***FURTHER ACTION,*** if any, is required, such as follow-up calls or a physical check-in.
» G2G "informs" on the user's location at all times. It communicates with adjacent smart devices (via Bluetooth, for example) to assess the ***INTERACTION*** between users, ***VICINITY*** between users, ***MOVEMENT*** between users ...
» In some embodiments, the app will also be used to send personal communication to the "target." Ex.: ***"COME AND BE VACCINATED."***
» Additional personalized communications might include a warning to avoid certain locations at high risk of contagion.

The G2G App launched at the beginning of October by Australian authorities is said to be a tool to help Western Australia police "protect" the community by conducting remote "virtual" app checks on people in quarantine. The G2G uses:

» Facial recognition technology
» Phone location data
» The user's registered address

This data is to ensure people in quarantine remain at their registered addresses throughout their quarantine periods. More disturbing details of this surveillance include:

- If you miss the "check-in" multiple times and do not provide a "valid" reason, ***POLICE MAY ATTEND YOUR ADDRESS TO CHECK ON YOUR QUARANTINE COMPLIANCE.***
- If you have traveled from a "high risk" area and you are over 16, you are legally required to comply with G2G Now App instructions.
- One who consistently fails to comply with check-in requests without a ***GOOD REASON*** may have committed ***AN OFFENSE*** under the Emergency Management Act. This can result in fines up to $50,000 and ***IMPRISONMENT***.
- Warning to those who "dissent," that G2G Now allows authorities to "individualize" people's check-in requirements.
  a. Some get "check-in" demands at different times of the day.
  b. Some get ***MORE THAN OTHER PEOPLE.***
- Photos of users are said to be kept by police only for monitoring quarantine, and not for general use. But it will be "stored and used as permitted or required by law."

Kingston commented, "Everything about you is now owned by the government. The WHO describes use of software to be incorporated to stop 'super spreaders.' Under the Obama Care Act, on December 13, 2016, Section 3024 was passed. This states that under a UA and under clinical research, ***'INFORMED CONSENT' IS WAIVED*** if 'informed consent' is ***'NOT IN THE BEST INTEREST OF A HUMAN SUBJECT TO KNOW.'*** So if our government decides we shouldn't know we were injected with a smart device, that it's not in our best interest, then that would not be disclosed to us."

Kingston informs us that a close association with these COVID apps and the coming push for A.I. (artificial intelligence) exists. Part of the U.S. commitment to the "Organization for Economic Cooperation and Development" is reflected in the ominous words of Lynne Parker, the director of the Artificial Intelligence Initiative at the White House: "We must prepare the future and present U.S. workforce for integration of A.I. systems across all sectors of the economy and society." This plan, Kingston explained, includes everything from kindergarten to community college and the eventual evil goal is to replace healthcare and other American workers with A.I.

[Perhaps significantly, LifeSiteNews, on the fifty-eighth anniversary of the JFK assassination (November 22, 2021), revealed this Nazi-like news. Pierre Boralevi had this headline:]

Australian army hauls 38 citizens to quarantine facility over some positive COVID tests

The group of 38, identified by health authorities as either positive cases or "close contacts," was taken in army trucks to Howard Springs quarantine facility, located at a former mining camp near Darwin in northern Australia.

DARWIN, Australia (LifeSiteNews)—The government of Australia's Northern Territory has ordered the transfer of 38 Australians from a remote Aboriginal town to a quarantine facility. Nine people there had tested positive for COVID-19. The group of 38, identified by health authorities as either positive cases or "close contacts," was taken in army trucks to Howard Springs quarantine facility, located at a former mining camp near Darwin in northern Australia. "It is highly likely that more residents will be transferred to Howard Springs today either as positive cases or close contacts," announced Michael Gunner, chief minister of the Northern Territory, at a press conference Sunday.

In the Aboriginal town of Binjari near Katherine, in Australia's Northern Territory, nine people tested positive for COVID. Both Binjari and the neighboring town of Rockhole are now fully locked down. Residents are not allowed to leave their homes except for emergencies, medical treatment, or "if required by law." Gunner described Binjari as a "low-vaccination community" but said the vaccination status of the positive cases "has not been confirmed yet." He also thanked the Australian armed forces for assisting with the transfer of positive cases and close contacts to the quarantine facility. "We are grateful for the support of about 20 ADF (Australian Defence Forces) personnel as well as army trucks to assist with the transfer of positive cases and close contacts and to support the communities," said Gunner.

According to the Northern Territory's official COVID website, there are two "mandatory supervised quarantine facilities" in that part of the country. One is located in Alice Springs, and the other, called the "Centre for National Resilience," in Howard Springs, just south of Darwin. According to engineering firm AECOM, the facility can host up to 850 people.

THE STUNNING FINAL HEAD OF THE SNAKE AUSTRALIA REALITY CHECK

Australia's COVID "vaccine" rollout was secretly headed up by the U.S. Military: report

(Ethan Huff, NaturalNews, January 13, 2023)

All that tyranny we told you about that took place in Australia throughout the COVID "pandemic" was headed up, secretly, by none other than the United States military. From the initial lockdowns to the mask and "vaccine" mandates, all of it was spearheaded by the U.S. Department of Defense (DoD), which embedded its people within the power structure of Australia in order to subdue the nation under tyranny and genocide. Pharmacologist Phillip Altman and a group of Australian scientists, doctors, and medical academics all claim that the DoD "had a dominant role in the response to the SARS-CoV-2 virus and in the subsequent development, manufacture, and distribution of the COVID-19 vaccines."

Operation Warp Speed allowed the DoD to manufacture the injections rapidly. Those injections were plunged into the arms of Aussies, many of whom had no choice but to comply—or else lose their livelihoods and ultimately their lives

All power Down Under was handed to the U.S. military-industrial complex. "... all decisions from that point onward to the present day were subject to full command and control from them.

["Danger, If Another 2025 'Plandemic' Comes," Michelle Malkin told Stew Peters, November 11, 2021:]

"***The Smart Health Card*** is now approved in five states and countless counties." The journalist points out, "There are taxpayers and parents who have no idea this system has been introduced. It's been in the works for years."

She explained there is a consortium of "big tech," "big pharma" and companies including ***Microsoft*** and ***Oracle***, and institutions, including Boston Children's Hospital. This "wolf in sheep's clothes" masquerades as a private non-profit consortium, but it has plenty of federal funding behind it. Malkin designated the V.C.I., ***"Vaccine Credential Initiative,"*** as the linchpin for this new, unprecedented surveillance system. "The V.C.I.," explains Malkin, "is how the Smart Health card is making the entire ***tracking*** and ***tracing*** system ***"interoperable."***

According to Malkin's research, this system's tentacles are already deeply imbedded in many of America's county health agencies and schools. Yes, parents, especially, have been electrified [to learn the Smart Health Card is in their school]. They are showing up at school board meetings. It is imperative all local residents must demand answers from their county health departments.

She concludes with this grave alert: "Look at Singapore as the example which initiated a health card and tracking system. ***V.C.I. AND THE SMART HEALTH CARD ARE A WAY OF TURNING ORDINARY CITIZENS, AND INDIVIDUALS, AND CERTAINLY ANY CHILDREN INTO LIFE-LONG QR CODES."***

—*compiled by Elizabeth Cuppett Caverly*

CHAPTER 23

2022—A Big Win!

GEORGIA STONES BROKEN, BUT WHEN WILL HEARTS BREAK—AND REPENT BEFORE GOD?

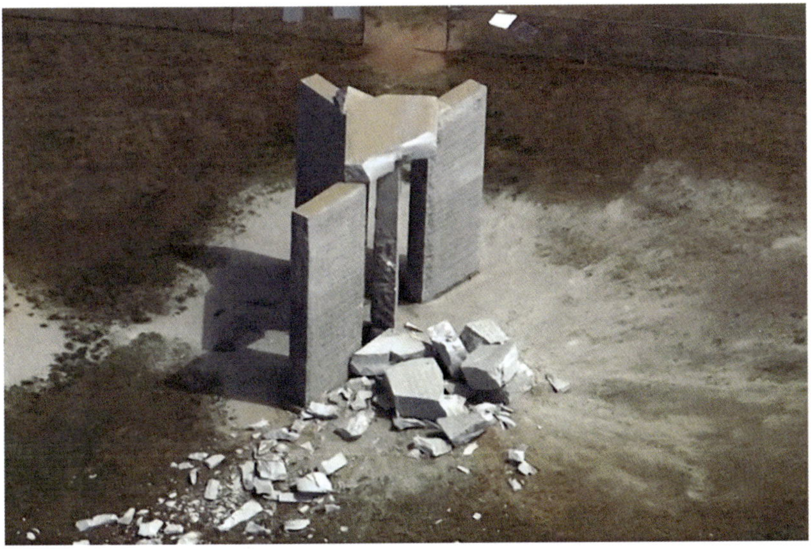

Many Americans felt spiritual joy at the news reported on July 7 that the Georgia Guidestones were attacked by demolition and then totally removed out of safety concerns. As one Divided Kingdom listener put it so well, "Nothing better with morning coffee to hear the Georgia Guidestones 'in rubble!' Arise, my 'American Republic Army,' to do battle ..."

The "American Stonehenge," with all its innuendoes (or direct connections) with human sacrifice is gone. Yet, the actual killing over the American heartland continues. Our hearts in this "heartland" are broken, our souls pierced by the latest mathematical documentation of iniquity. The abomination to Almighty God of casting our youngest babes, even six-month-olds to the devastation and devouring of the Molech mRNA COVID shots. This, even as political high priestesses sing "Happy Birthday" to masked 3-year-olds on-site at vaccine clinics. The First Lady said, "The relief is finally here—a vaccine for the youngest children."

LifeSiteNews reports, June 20, 2022, "Vatican City has issued a new set of coins, one of which shows a young person being vaccinated, presumably against COVID-19. The (20 Euro silver) coin does not specify the jab is for COVID, but LifeSite quotes from a Vatican website the following:

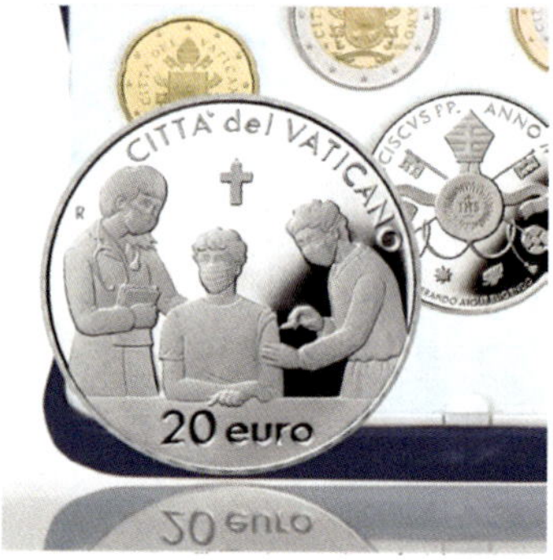

> The 20-euro silver coin designed by Chiara Principe, is dedicated to a current theme that is very close to Pope Francis' heart: treatments to counter the pandemic and the need to be vaccinated. The coin depicts a doctor, a nurse, and a young person who is ready to receive the vaccine. The Holy Father has repeatedly stressed the importance of vaccination, recalling that health care is 'a moral obligation,' and it is important to 'continue efforts to immunize even the poorest people.'"

Yes, the poorest peoples, the dark-skinned races, those with mental or physical handicaps, and the elderly, all must receive priority. The Guidestones' abominably murderous words in the dusty air of its death: its first commandment—"Keep the earth's population in balance at 500 million ..."

Has God called Christian men and women to "stand in the gap"? Who will answer with courage and truth about the COVID bioweapon world genocide? Probably not the world's leading religious figures, as we earlier noted: Dr. Franklin Graham ("What would Jesus do?"), Dr. Gordon Robertson, Albert Mohler, Pope Francis, and others.

How about the smaller churches in America? Talk to your church and business friends who got the shots. Especially the ones who then got COVID, itself. The dialogue might go something like this:

"Did your pastor warn you about the abortion-derived COVID shots?

"No, my pastor never said anything about it."

The shepherds were silent. Was it their ignorance? Greed? Cowardice? All three? May God raise up new godly pastor warriors. Events worse than millstone-around-the-neck drownings await the others. Blood on the hands of the guilty and the silent.

Repent, Oh Church!

—Elizabeth Cuppett Caverly

CHAPTER 24

2022—A Loss!

BLEEDING KANSAS

From 1850 to 2022, has a demonic Molech stronghold of blood and sacrifice been holding the state of Kansas captive?

Roe v. Wade has now been reversed, and every state must decide where it stands on the subject of abortion. Some states, like Missouri, have already enacted laws (or reactivated earlier laws that are still in force) to ban abortions or severely restrict them. Others, like California and New York, have promised to allow abortions almost without limit. Kansas is a special case, since it will require an amendment to the Kansas state constitution to restrict abortions in that state. Kansas voters will be the first in the nation to cast votes on abortion rights.

This called to mind events in that same region of the United States 168 years ago. At that time, in 1854, slavery was an issue that had been threatening to tear the country apart for at least a half-century. The Missouri Compromise of 1820 admitted Maine to the Union as a free state and Missouri as a slave state. Slavery was prohibited in the region of the Louisiana Purchase north of latitude 33° 30', a line which ran along Missouri's southern border. This cooled tempers somewhat and remained in force for over thirty years. Thomas Jefferson wrote to a friend, "The Missouri question ... filled me with terror. I considered it the death knell of the Union. It is hushed indeed for the moment. But this is a reprieve only, not a final sentence."

During the next four decades, new regions had been settled in the west. By the 1850s, Kansas was among those areas ready to become U.S. territories, as was Nebraska. Once again, the issue of slavery sharply divided the nation. The balance between pro-slavery and anti-slavery members of the U.S. Senate was at stake. In 1854 the Kansas-Nebraska Act became law in spite of intense opposition. It repealed the Missouri Compromise and provided for both Kansas and Nebraska to settle the slavery question by a vote of the citizens of that territory, not by the United States Congress—hence the name "popular sovereignty."

On the surface, that seemed a reasonable solution. However, the balance of power in the United States Senate could be tipped by the outcome of the vote in Kansas. Both sides of the slavery issue decided action was needed. Within a short time, outsiders flooded into Kansas to try to sway the vote to favor or oppose slavery. "Border ruffians" from the South invaded the state and "Free-Staters" from the North did the same.

Violence broke out in the territory. Homes and barns were burned, people were beaten and a number were killed. Border ruffians attacked the city of Lawrence, Kansas. In response, abolitionist John Brown and seven followers killed five men at Pottawatomie Creek in May of 1856. Horace Greeley, editor of the *New York Tribune,* coined the term "Bleeding Kansas." In December of 1859, just before he was hanged for treason following his unsuccessful raid on the U.S. arsenal at Harper's Ferry, Brown uttered these prophetic words: "I, John Brown, am now quite certain that the crimes of this guilty land will never be purged away, but with Blood." In less than two years, his words had come true. The Civil War had begun.

Now, in 2022, Horace Greeley's term, "Bleeding Kansas," once again puts the national spotlight on that state's "Molech" murder-stronghold. This time the controversy is not slavery, but abortion. In the wake of the repeal of *Roe v. Wade* by the U.S. Supreme Court, no doubt most citizens in Kansas would like to limit abortions there. After *Roe v. Wade* went into effect in 1973, demonic leftists in the Kansas Supreme Court declared their anti-abortion laws unconstitutional. They were nullified. In contrast, Missouri can immediately enforce its prior existing anti-abortion laws. The people of Kansas votes on August 2 on an amendment to their constitution to reinstate anti-abortion laws. Until the August 2 vote, there is no law in place to restrict any woman in the state from having an abortion.

"Bleeding Kansas" abortion vacation? The Kansas vote will have regional and national implications. Failure to pass the amendment could make Kansas an abortion sanctuary for women from Missouri and other restricting states. Just as in 1854, the stakes are high. Those in favor of a "yes" vote on August 2 to adopt the new amendment have formed the "Value Them Both Coalition" (VTB). The name of the proposed amendment is also "Value Them Both."

VTB warns that failure to pass "Value Them Both" will change the state into another New York or California. The sacrifice of infants to the fires of Satan will proliferate. In addition, most hideous of all, late-term abortions may become widespread in Kansas.

Just as in the slavery divide, both sides of the abortion debate are passionate. Neither side is about to compromise. We may not see the kind of viciousness that characterized Kansas from 1854 until the end of the Civil War. Yet attacks on churches and pro-life centers have already begun. Extremist groups are enraged at the SCOTUS decision. Federal marshals had to guard some of the justices from assassination before the ruling took place. Some crazed leftists are still advocating violence against them.

Once again, as in the 1850s, the "Bleeding Kansas" stronghold is at the climactic center of the war between God and Satan. The voters of Kansas have a chance to break that demonic grip on August 2. The late evangelist Henry Gruver spent much of his life visiting many countries around the world. His goal was to walk around cities praying for God to destroy Luciferian control. Not just Kansas, but the whole U.S.A., needs all of our prayers, the kind of prayers Gruver made to God—to reclaim our entire country. This can happen only after a spirit of deep repentance convicts every person in the land. Then, God's renewal and restoration can come once more to America.

•••

In August 2023, this researcher checked on the present status of things in Kansas and found:

- On August 2, 2022, an amendment to the Kansas constitution was defeated by a margin of approximately 60 to 40. The amendment would have prohibited abortions in the state.
- The state currently has a few very mild restrictions on getting an abortion. For example, there is a 24-hour waiting period. Only the most radical abortion proponents could object to this very slight requirement.
- The woman must also receive counseling and view an ultrasound of her developing fetus. A similar rule would apply in the case of any serious operation, even something as routine as gall bladder surgery. Of course, abortion providers try to portray this as highly out-of-the ordinary.

These abortion requirements are so basic and easy to fulfill, one gets the impression they were adopted merely to "put on a good show." ***Kansas is still bleeding!***

—Lou Caverly

BOOK TWO

NWO CHAOS COMMENCES

CHAPTER TWENTY-FIVE

Two Continuing Concerns: Pandemic Treaty and Pilots

April 21, 2022, Maria Zee was interviewed on Brighteon.com. Maria reported on a meeting the World Health Organization held with representatives of many nations. The topic was a proposed pandemic treaty. If ratified by 70 percent of the world's countries, this treaty would result in the WHO taking control of all responses to a future pandemic. This could include FORCED VACCINATION! According to the U.S. Constitution, any treaty must be ratified by the U.S. Senate. Of course, this administration would try to bypass that requirement. We must not let that happen. This treaty, as we state elsewhere in this book, failed to be ratified in the spring of 2023. In 2024 and onward, we must watch out for this sinister nemesis to return.

Maria explains that this is all about bringing in one-world government. The city of Newcastle, Australia, has become a model "Smart City." It reminds one of dystopian cities found in movies. The authorities will have no problem spying on every resident. 5G towers will be placed at every street corner. Australia is the prototype for world government.

The other great concern is many sick pilots, a frightening danger to all Americans using air travel. Mandatory vaccine policies of major American airlines have created it. A number of pilots have become seriously ill from the shots, some even while flying. Months ago, a Delta Airlines pilot suffered a post-COVID shot sudden cardiovascular collapse while landing. Fortunately for the passengers, the co-pilot was able to safely bring the plane in. Delta at first denied the incident, but word of it spread everywhere.

This Delta near-tragedy was not an anomaly. On April 9, Captain Robert Snow suffered cardiac arrest within one minute of landing his American Airlines Denver-to-Dallas Flight #1067. Medics did CPR on him and shocked his heart three times to bring him back. A special high-profile team from Baylor University was assembled. The team included Dr. Peter McCullough and Lt. Col. Dr. Teresa Long. Two hundred people were on the plane. If his heart attack had come just six minutes earlier, all of those lives could have been lost. Once again, this story was covered up.

Advocate and whistleblower Joshua Yoder of U.S. Freedom Flyers, as Stew Peter's April 18 guest, quoted one pilot as saying, "American Airlines coerced me into getting the shot." Yoder also reported that Captain Snow had no prior adverse health conditions. He also described the case of a flight attendant who suffered four strokes after getting the COVID shots. She told Yoder that she didn't think she'd live much longer. This danger is far from over.

Newspunch.com, March 15, 2023, reported:

> **United Airlines Plane Makes Emergency Landing after Fully-Vaxxed Pilot Suffers Heart Attack Mid-flight**
>
> A United Airlines Flight from Guatemala to Chicago was force to divert to Houston International Airport after the pilot suffered an apparent heart attack mid-flight and became incapacitated, sparking concern among passengers.

America (and for that matter, the world) of today is in crisis. This is creeping (or sometimes zooming) in upon us. If we do not raise our voices and fight back, we will lose our lives. Or if not our lives, the future will be worse than Orwell's *1984* ever was.

—*Elizabeth Cuppett Caverly*

CHAPTER TWENTY-SIX

Short-Take Excerpt: U.S. Planned for Our Starvation Years

PLANNED FAMINE:
U.S. government has been paying farmers to destroy crops and livestock for years

(Ethan Huff, on NaturalNews.com)

Listening to the "news" these days, one is led to believe that everything is falling apart economically and agriculturally because Russia invaded Ukraine. The truth, however, is that this engineered takedown of the global economy began many years ago and is only now becoming visible.

Two years ago when the Wuhan coronavirus (COVID-19) *plandemic* was launched, it was being reported that the United States government was quietly paying farmers to destroy their own crops and depopulate livestock. Watch the video from *Brighteon.com*. This video is from the channel "Freedom."

This was reiterated again about a year ago when actual farmers started sharing videos on social media about how the food supply was being tampered with by government officials. This video is from the channel "Warrior68" on Brighteon.com.

If your family goes hungry, ask your government why it destroyed the food supply with your tax dollars. It would appear as though the plan all along was to quietly start throwing a few wrenches into the supply chain at that time to get the ball rolling. It was easy to blame the resulting problems on "COVID," and this continued for a full two years. As the two-year anniversary of the plandemic approached, things got increasingly more chaotic. And now we have reached a point of no return, it seems, which is why the narrative shifted from COVID to Vladimir Putin.

The timing of Russia's invasion of Ukraine is suspect because it occurred just as the consequences of several years of *planned and engineered famine* were really starting to become apparent. This provided cover for the media to blame Putin for even higher gas and food prices and the coming prospect of global food shortages. For the past month, we have been told that because of the invasion and associated sanctions, natural gas is now in short supply. Natural gas, it turns out, is used to produce the fertilizer for food crops. *It is almost as if somebody wants food to become scarce so that the people become easier to control* [emphasis added]. With Putin as the new fall guy (it was COVID prior to this), the next engineered phase of the global plandemic can simply be blamed on Russia.

You may recall that we reported numerous times in years past about bad weather conditions that interfered with crop yields. We warned that in the future, these losses would catch up with the supply chain and cause problems.

What we did not know at the time was that a *plandemic* was going to be launched to create a "perfect storm"-type of situation in which the dominoes would begin to fall more quickly and more severely, creating confusion as to the cause.

This is how the powers that be are keeping all eyes off of themselves. *They launch chaos event after chaos event while quietly knocking over the dominoes on purpose in the background undetected.*

Watch the two videos above and ask yourself: Why did the American government use American tax dollars to destroy precious food resources? And how is it impacting the world now as the very real prospect of mass starvation looms over the world?

"If we do not hang together against this murderous takeover, we WILL hang separately!" wrote someone at Brighteon.com. ***"Opposing this as a***

majority is our only hope. *If we do not stand up together, they will put us down for good."*

More related news about the engineered destruction of the old-world order can be found at Conspiracy.news.

—Lou Caverly

CHAPTER TWENTY-SEVEN

Poison Food

Right around the time Lou and I began our radio work in 2003, a controversy about EU revolutionary new food regulations erupted. "Codex Alimentarius," a set of bizarre requirements, set the stage for coming harmful adulteration to our food supply in the decades ahead. Chemicals and quotients of substances not good for the body were required as additives.

If we recall correctly, it was Augusto Perez, a prophetic man of God, who said that in a dream or vision, he saw the future. There was plenty of food on the grocery shelves, no scarcity. But all the food he saw was *poisoned, toxic.*

In this context, in spring 2023, a diabolical change in meat regulations threatened. This Sword of Damocles hung over all of us. An excerpt from a special April 7, 2023 Infowars report warns:[8]

> The UK recently passed into law the Genetic Technology Precision Breeding Bill. The Bill amends the Environmental Protection Act of 1990 to exclude references to precision-bred organisms so far as they relate to marketing.
>
> "Precision-bred organism" is another term for gene-edited. So now in the UK, food that's been gene-edited can be legally marketed as non-GMO, and if this UK gene-edited meat makes its way to America, it can be labeled non-GMO here as well, and so long as it's butchered in America, it can be labeled "Product of USA."
>
> The fake alternative meat being pushed by Bill Gates and others

> is made of immortal cell lines. In other words, cancerous tumor cells. Real meat is being blamed for climate change. And a recent independent study suggests that most of our meat is already contaminated.
>
> Using infrared spectroscopy and electron microscopy, Dr. Ana Maria Mihalcea has been studying the blood of the vaxxed and the unvaxxed for over a year now. And at first, she was finding the same contamination in only the blood of the vaxxed, a contamination that she describes as "ribbon-like structures," much like the mysterious blood clots being found by coroners. But lately she's been finding these ribbon-like structures in the blood of the unvaxxed as well.
>
> By measuring the frequency of one of these mysterious, rubbery blood clots, Dr. David Jernigan has developed a way of detecting the same frequency in the vaxxed. Recently, he's found this unique frequency in the meat being sold in his local grocery store and asked Dr. Mihalcea to confirm his findings. Her microscopy showed that the blood samples taken from products in the grocery store were all contaminated with the similar ribbon-like structures found in the blood of the vaxxed.
>
> Most of the meat in the grocery store is from overseas, and if we want to eat uncontaminated meat, we'll have to start buying direct from farms in America that still produce all-natural organic protein and take back control of our democidal government.

This awful change to our beef was finally supposed to commence at the beginning of August. All the voices of America who vociferously opposed this became a winning crescendo. The Cattlemen's and Pork Associations dropped the idea! We had heard reports that pork production had already been using some mRNA vaccines for some time. It is hard to verify whether or not that has been the case.

One thing we can verify—that very ominous lab work is going on to change meat and also plants.

Here is an excerpt that provokes great concern, from an article entitled "FDA SAYS CRISPR GENE EDITED cattle safe for human consumption."

Cattle created using CRISPR Gene Editing produced by Acciligen, have been declared safe for human consumption by the FDA.

The United States Food and Drug Administration (FDA) has ruled that short-haired cattle created using CRISPR gene-editing technology are safe to eat. The PRLR-SLICK calves were the first to earn an FDA "low-risk determination for enforcement discretion" after the agency found that the two genome-edited bovine's intentional genomic alteration (IGA) does not pose any safety risks.

The cows, developed by Acciligen with climate change in mind, have a genetic feature that gives them a short, sleek coat that is supposed to assist the animals cope better with hot temperatures. Because of the FDA's low-risk decision, Acciligen, a "precision breeding" company, is unlikely to seek regulatory permission before releasing cattle products.

According to the company website, the majority of Acceligen's employees have agricultural backgrounds. Precision breeding, according to the company, differs from conventional breeding and genetically modified organisms (GMOs) in that it permits a "highly desired trait" to be produced in "just one breeding cycle," as opposed to years.

Acceligen, a Recombinetics Inc. firm, stated in 2020 that it had obtained a $3.68 million grant from the Bill and Melinda Gates Foundation to create bovine genetics with desirable qualities for smallholder dairy farmers in SSA dairy systems. A "suite of traits" from the breeding program's discovery pipeline will be introduced into commercially relevant dairy animals "with high genetic merit for production and durability." The grant's project lead, Tad Sonstegard, CEO of Acceligen, stated of the endeavor:

"When we combine gene editing with top merit animals using advanced reproductive technologies from our partners Kheiron (Pilar, Argentina) and TransOva Genetics (Sioux Center, Iowa), we can make significant genetic improvement for well-adapted, high yielding dairy cows. Our goal is to get these animals into the hands of smallholder farmers."

CRISPR has been used to create disease-resistant chickens and pigs, as well as mosquitos that are unable to bite or produce eggs, according to researchers. They're also working on a number of projects, such as developing disease-resistant crops, such as grapes for winemaking. They're also working on genetically modifying pigs so that their organs can be transplanted into people.

A 57-year-old man was on the verge of death when he received a genetically altered pig heart in January, the first between-species transplant that had been "hailed as a success" through xenotransplantation, the technique of transporting tissues between species. The individual, however, began to deteriorate roughly 40 days after the transplant, and he died two months later. "No obvious cause identified at the time of his death," the hospital said at first. Despite this, the patient's heart was infected with a pig virus, according to *MIT Technology Review* on May 4. MIT wrote on the complex process:

The biggest obstacle to animal-organ transplants is the human immune system, which ferociously attacks foreign cells in a process called rejection. To avoid rejection, companies have been engineering pigs—removing some genes and adding others—to give their tissue a stealth profile that hides from immune attack.

Transferring pig viruses to humans has been a worry—some fear xenotransplantation could set off a pandemic if a virus were to adapt inside a patient's body and then spread to doctors and nurses. The concern could be serious enough to require lifelong monitoring for patients.

According to *Scientific America*, the first clinical experiments injecting CRISPR directly into living humans began in 2020, with the goal of correcting a genetic abnormality that causes blindness.

While CRISPR "reliably cuts DNA where we want it to," new research have proven that it can also alter genes that aren't on the target list. Even if we could get it to operate consistently, several experts have raised ethical concerns about utilizing the technology for eugenics and "designer babies," as *SA* points out. "If one day parents can pay scientists to edit their babies' DNA to make them stronger and smarter, CRISPR might make the world even more unequal and prejudiced," *SA* said. *SA* claims that, considering the risks of modifying the human genome, researchers are still a long way from using

CRISPR in medicine on a large scale, adding:

"CRISPR has given science a tool to reliably tinker with the code of life. But the question remains: can we do so safely and ethically while avoiding the unintended consequences of such power?"

The FDA took years to evaluate the two other genetically modified animals allowed for human consumption: a faster-growing salmon and a pig that the agency found was safe for those with meat allergies to eat. The FDA highlighted that gene-editing results in the same slick-hair feature seen in cattle in conventional agriculture, therefore the review process for the CRISPR beef cattle took less than a year. Steven Solomon, director of the FDA Center for Veterinary Medicine, remarked of the approval on March 7, 2022:

"We expect that our decision will encourage other developers to bring animal biotechnology products forward for the FDA's risk determination in this rapidly developing field, paving the way for animals containing low-risk IGAs (intentional genomic alterations) to more efficiently reach the marketplace."

There is no definite timeline for when CRISPR cow beef will be available in U.S. supermarkets, but it might be as soon as two years. It's also uncertain whether the meat from gene-edited cows will be labeled differently from regular beef.

[In addition, Dr. Joseph Mercola, LifeSite News, June 24, 2022 said, "The GMO industry is seeking to replace beef, poultry, dairy, and fish with synthetic biology, cultured meat, precision fermentation, cellular-based and gene-edited foods." Mercola explains that cultured meat for control of the masses is a Great Reset goal. Mercola explains: "Cultured meat (cell-based meat) is produced from animal tissue cells that are grown in fetal bovine serum (FBS) made from the blood of both cows and unborn calves which are drained of their blood while still alive. **Gruesome!**]

Plants are not free either from being mixed with dangerous elements. [Can anyone say COVID-19 vaccine elements?!!] So, we must warn you about coming dangers in both plants and animals in our food supply. Once again, the April 2022 special report explains:

The genetic editing of plants to contain edible vaccines is well underway. Work is being done with bananas, potatoes, tomatoes, lettuce, rice, wheat, soybeans, and corn. Companies like Medicago are using gene editing to turn plants into mini-bioreactors.

News Clip: "Medicago's manufacturing facility looks like a nursery, but inside these plants, they're growing a new kind of vaccine. The technology is called a virus-like-particle ..."

Promo Video: "At Medicago, we use a careful step-by-step process to develop vaccines using our plants as mini-bioreactors. We start with the gene sequence or code of a virus. We then use our technology to synthesize the virus code into a real biological product. The code contains genetic instructions that our plants can read, and we insert it into bacteria called *Agrobacterium tumefaciens.*

"We submerge the plants in a bath with the bacteria that carries the information into the plant cells and using a vacuum, we suck out the air between the plant cells and replace it with the liquid. The plants absorb it like a sponge. At the end of their bacterial bath, we return our plants to a carefully controlled greenhouse to let them get on with our natural growing business for at least four days. Now, the plants will start producing the most important ingredient of our vaccines: virus-like-particles."

—*compiled by Elizabeth Cuppett Caverly*

CHAPTER TWENTY-EIGHT

Beyond Meat and More

Check out the NASTY ingredients in Beyond Meat burgers
(Ethan Huff, *Natural News*, Monday, October 24, 2022)

[The kind of food you readers find right now in your grocery stores has to be put under much deeper scrutiny than years back. Plant-based substitutes for real foods are proliferating everywhere. We are printing a large excerpt from this article to help you.]

> If you have ever wondered what, exactly, is contained within Beyond Meat's fake "meat" burger patties, look no further than the following list of the top-most toxic ingredients:
>
> **Pea protein isolate:** While one of the few ingredients that is not genetically modified (GMO), pea protein isolate constitutes much of the bulk matter used to create Beyond Meat patties.
>
> Pea protein isolate is problematic for many because it is an allergen. It is also linked to reduced kidney function, containing a substance class known as purines that convert to uric acid.
>
> "While purines aren't bad in normal amounts, excess doses could make it difficult for your kidneys to get rid of all the uric acid," it is explained.
>
> "This increases the risk of gout, an inflammatory condition in which uric acid builds up in the blood, creating needle-like crystals in the joints that cause episodes of severe, sudden pain and tenderness." (Related: Learn more about the rise and fall of Beyond Meat.)

Canola oil: A common ingredient used in processed foods, canola oil is more often than not GMO. It is also an unhealthy, highly refined, omega-6 fatty acid-rich saturation of chemicals that does no favors for the body when consumed.

Another toxic ingredient in Beyond Meat patties is **DHA algal oil,** a substance known to cause gastrointestinal upset. DHA algal oil is often produced using a harsh and caustic chemical solvent called hexane.

"Hexane is a known neurotoxin (according to the Centers for Disease Control and Prevention) and hazardous air pollutant (according to the Environmental Protection Agency)," reports indicate. "The use of hexane is strictly prohibited in organic food production."

DHA algal oil is also typically stabilized and preserved using *synthetic* chemicals that are prohibited, including the sugar alcohol mannitol, modified starch, glucose syrup solids, and ascorbyl palmitate.

Methylcellulose: This natural plant substance is linked to allergic reactions such as hives, breathing problems, face and lip swelling, and other symptoms. It can also cause stomach cramps, rectal bleeding, and an impacted bowel.

Carrageenan: A pseudo-latex substance derived from seaweed, carrageenan causes many of the same allergic symptoms as actual latex. Its consumption is linked to large bowel ulceration and ulcerative colitis, fetal toxicity and birth defects, colorectal and liver cancer, glucose intolerance and insulin resistance, inflammation, immune suppression, and the growth of abnormal colon glands.

Yeast extract: Another name for monosodium glutamate (MSG), yeast extract causes many of the same symptoms as MSG including flushing of the skin and headaches.

"Too much glutamate in abnormally high concentrations can lead to overexcitation of the receiving nerve cell. In some cases, the nerve cell receptors for glutamate can be oversensitive, and fewer molecules are necessary to excite that cell," the science says. (See sources below.)

"The ALS Association says prolonged excitation is toxic to nerve cells, and glutamate can cause harm when the messages are overwhelming, as in stroke or epilepsy."

Maltodextrin: Usually extracted from potatoes, rice, or GMO corn, maltodextrin has a higher glycemic index than table sugar, which is a disaster for diabetics. This ingredient also damages the balance of gut bacteria, which play an important role in immune regulation.

"One study has shown that maltodextrin increases the activity of *Escherichia coli* (E. coli) bacteria, which is linked to inflammatory bowel diseases and other intestinal damage."

More related news about Beyond Meat and other fake "meat" companies can be found at Frankenfood.news.

—*compiled by Lou Caverly*

CHAPTER TWENTY-NINE

Global Food Supply—Sabotage, Control, and Coming Famine

"Control of food production will guarantee massive genocide"

—Kelleigh Nelson

[Excerpts from a remarkably cogent essay follow:]

(Kelleigh Nelson, "The Global Food System and Totalitarian Control," July 19, 2022)

Klaus Schwab, Founder and Executive Chairman, World Economic Forum, made it clear when he said, "The pandemic represents a rare but narrow window of opportunity to reflect, reimagine and reset our world."

There's only one conclusion, they want us dead. Those who survive will be enslaved.

Control of food production will guarantee massive genocide.

Blackrock, Vanguard, and State Street

In August of 2021, Jim O'Neill wrote a stunning expose of Blackrock, Vanguard, and State Street entitled "Monolithic Monopoly." Take a gander at it. Jim has listed the large companies of which Vanguard, Blackrock, and State Street are top shareholders. His article first alerted me to Blackrock's Chairman and CEO, Larry Fink.

In March of 2022, Investopedia reported, "BlackRock Inc. (BLK) is by some measures the biggest investment management company across the globe, with more than $10.0 trillion in assets under management (AUM) as of Dec. 31, 2021. [9] As a major publicly traded company with a market capitalization of about $112.3 billion, Black Rock provides investment and technology services to both institutional and retail clients around the world."

According to a May 1, 2022 *Newstarget* article, Blackrock and Vanguard have taken over centralized food production technologies and will have near-total control over the future food supply in America. It's been under the radar for the majority of America, and it certainly doesn't bode well for the future. Remember Kissinger's famous quote, "Who controls the food supply controls the people; who controls the energy can control whole continents; who controls money can control the world."

The USDA and FDA have already approved lab-grown meat, genetically modified cattle, and are funding the globalists to research and develop cellular agriculture as well as indoor growers and genetics companies, while they slack on regulations for gene-edited produce.

Union Pacific is mandating railroad shipping reductions by 20%, impacting CF Industries Holdings, the world's largest fertilizer company. Vanguard, BlackRock, and State Street happen to be the top shareholders of Union Pacific, and BlackRock and Vanguard are in the top 3 shareholders of CF Industries Holdings.

Only 10 companies control almost every food and beverage brand in the world. Vanguard and Blackrock are the top shareholders in most of these companies. Their plans include owning all the seeds, produce, and meat. Everything will be grown inside secured facilities after a gene splice or inside a petri dish, and farmland will become dormant due to overreaching regulations, lack of supplies, and manufactured inflation.

No more farmer's markets.

Think we're kidding?! Over 100 food processing plants have caught fire and been destroyed. Conspiracy theory? Hardly!

Vertical Farming

Bill Gates owns tons of our farmland, 242,000 acres, but insists that all foods will eventually be grown in huge indoor vertical farming and will be in urban areas where people will migrate to, more like forced into. Who gets to sit at the table with healthy produce served up by Gates while the rest of the population eats gene-edited produce from locked-down facilities, delivered to their local grocery store, and accessed only through a digital ID? Check out the 11-minute video of one of these farms in Wyoming.

But guess what else Gates owns? In an April 27, 2022, article on controlled food systems, we read, "The Consultative Group of International Agriculture Research (CGIAR) holds the world's largest private seed banks consisting of 10% of the worldwide germplasm across the globe, which is controlled by the Bill & Melinda Gates Foundation, Rockefeller and Ford Foundations, and World Bank, managing 768,576 accessions of hijacked farmers seeds." How lovely! Total control by total evil!

In one of Dr. Joseph Mercola's articles, he stated the following:

"In August 2020, Monsanto/Bayer helped found a startup called Unfold, which develops new vegetable seed varieties specifically geared for vertical farms. According to investigative journalist, Corey Lynn, 'GMOs already account for 75 to 80% of food Americans consume,' and once fresh produce is under patent, that percentage will inch closer to 100%.

"The University of California is also working on plant-based mRNA vaccines. The idea there is to disseminate vaccines through the conventional food supply, which puts a whole new spin on the old adage to 'Let thy food be thy medicine.'" (Oh yummy!)

Good old Monsanto/Bayer who has allegedly poisoned the planet with Roundup's cancer-causing glyphosate has a long and evil history. Eva Moses Kor and her twin were in Auschwitz. Mrs. Kor sued Bayer and stated, "They were right there with Dr. Joseph Mengele at Auschwitz." The parties negotiated a settlement establishing the creation of a $5 billion fund for the Foundation Remembrance, Responsibility, and Future. I was fortunate to have had a lengthy conversation with Eva in 1997; what an unbelievably amazing woman.

German companies, Bayer and BASF, two of the world's largest suppliers of seed, are both heavily involved with the vertical farm industry.

It was during the Obama administration in 2014 when congress established the Foundation for Food and Agriculture Research Act (FFAR) through the Farm Bill, which ultimately created a non-profit organization outside of the government with a $200 million kickoff from taxpayer dollars and additional millions in support from Bill Gates as seen here, and here. Then a 15-member board of directors was appointed which unsurprisingly included deputy director Dr. Robert Horsch of the Bill & Melinda Gates Foundation and high-ranking employees from Cargill and the Aspen Institute, among others.

In March of 2020, America was locked down due to COVID. We lost many of our unalienable rights, especially those of the First Amendment. That summer, Antifa and Black Lives Matter looted and torched the entire country.

America was set ablaze, but the Insurrection Act was never used. There were no mayors like Richard J. Daley.

Communism isn't on its way, it's already here.

Klaus Schwab wants to "reflect, reimagine and reset our world."

Yes, a reset to totalitarian control. The world population and all its resources will be run by governments empowered to "fairly" distribute goods and services to the people.

Food production is the number one target of control by the World Economic Forum's Great Reset. The key to genocide is food control and a totalitarian slave system.

As Americans, we must make Schwab's "rare but narrow window" an impossibility.

Kelleigh Nelson has been researching the Christian right, the New Age, and cults since 1975. Formerly an executive producer for three different national radio talk show hosts, Kelleigh was born and raised in Chicago, Illinois. She was a Goldwater girl with high school classmate Hillary Rodham in Park Ridge, Illinois.

—*compiled by Lou and Elizabeth Caverly*

CHAPTER THIRTY

Poultry & Pigs Killed by Strange Fires; American Food Plants Destroyed

FOOD PROCESSING PLANT FIRES: CONSPIRACY OR COINCIDENCE?

The Western Standard has been following the story closely and found dozens upon dozens of incidents globally.[10]

The outlet recapped some of the more recent incidents, which it compiled in this list (this is only a partial list, TWS's full list is here—https://westernstandardonline.com/2022/04/exclusive-destruction-of-food-plants-a-global-phenomenon/):

- On Monday, 43,000 chickens died in a massive fire that destroyed four chicken houses on a farm in the Dutch town of Heusden, according to *World Today News.*
- In March, a fire at a poultry farm in India killed 3,500 chickens. According to *PiPa News,* the fire destroyed the entire farm.
- Another poultry farm in India was also hit by fire in March killing 8,500 chicks. *Times of India* reported the fire may have been caused by a short circuit.
- In January, a fire at a poultry farm in Kerala, India, killed more than 2,500 chickens, according to *The Print.*
- In December 2021, 8,000 chickens were killed in a poultry farm blaze in Sri Lanka. *News First* reported the fire was likely sparked by an "electrical leak."

- » A massive blaze at a Northern Ireland farm killed hundreds of pigs in November 2021, as reported by *News Letter.* No one was injured.
- » In October 2021, a large fire at a Fermanagh poultry farm in Northern Ireland killed 16,000 birds. It took firefighters more than seven hours to get control of the fire, as reported by *That's Farming.*
- » A large fire broke out in September 2021 at a Chilean food processing plant. Although no injuries were reported, several crews were needed to battle the blaze, as reported by *La Tercera.*
- » In July 2021, a deadly fire at a Bangladesh food processing factory kills at least 52 people, as reported by *Al Jazeera.*
- » Another fire at a poultry house in East Yorkshire, England, in July 2021 killed 50,000 chickens. The fire was said to be caused by accidental ignition, as reported by the *Daily Mail.*
- » In April 2021, over 55,000 pigs were killed after a fire broke out at a German pig farm. *USA Today* reported the cause of the blaze was unclear.

In addition to a large number of blazes all over the world that killed thousands of animals, here is a list encompassing suspect explosions and accidents targeting food-processing and fertilizer plants across America.

- » Fayetteville, Illinois—1/15/21: Deli Star deals with the aftermath of devastating fire
- » Hanceville, Alabama—7/30/21: Tyson poultry meal plant suffered total loss in large fire
- » Scott Township, Pennsylvania—11/29/21: Seventeen departments fight fire at Maid-Rite Steak Co. meat processing plant
- » Winston-Salem, North Carolina—1/31/22: Thousands flee homes near Winston-Salem fertilizer plant fire
- » Mauston, Wisconsin—2/3/22: Portion of Wisconsin River Meats a "total loss" in overnight fire
- » Claypool, Indiana—2/16/22: Louis Dreyfus reports fire at largest U.S. soy processing plant

» Hermiston, Oregon—2/22/22: Seven injured in explosion as fire engulfs Shearer's foods plant
» Lincoln, Nebraska—3/1/22: Shadow Brook Farm and Dutch Girl Creamery cheesemaking facility gutted by fire
» Sunnyside, Washington—3/1/22: Washington fertilizer plant fire forces evacuations
» Plainfield, Indiana—3/18/22: ATF begins on-site investigation into Walmart facility fire in Plainfield
» Jonesboro, Arkansas—3/22/22: Nestle Hot Pockets plant remains shuttered following fire
» Belfast, Maine—3/24/22: Crews respond to fire at Belfast potato processing plant
» Maricopa, Arizona—3/29/22: 50,000 lbs. of food destroyed after fire ripped through Maricopa food pantry
» San Juan, Texas—3/31/22: Rio Fresh's onion warehouse damaged in fire
» Conway, New Hampshire—4/12/22: Crews battled fire for sixteen hours at East Conway Beef and Pork
» Heyburn, Idaho—4/14/22: Plane crashes into Idaho potato and food processing plant, killing the pilot
» Salinas, California—4/14/22: Taylor Farms building is a "total loss" after large fire
» Dufur, Oregon—4/19/22: Fire destroys Azure Standard headquarter facility
» Leoti, Kansas—4/19/22: Fertilizer plant fire causes evacuations in western Kansas
» Covington, Georgia—4/22/22: Investigators comb through plane crash wreckage at General Mills plant in Covington
» Cedar Rapids, Iowa—4/23/22: Firefighters attack overnight flames at General Mills from the roof
» Lecompte, Louisiana—4/26/22: Explosion and fire reported at Cargill-Nutrena feed mill

More from the article's commentor:

Most of these are not paltry fires, but catastrophic infernos with flames visible from satellites and which often require thousands of nearby residents to evacuate. The losses are not being measured in the millions, but billions of dollars, and they all put more of America›s food supply under strain.

One such accident is a tragedy. Two is an oddity. Three is a coincidence. But dozens? That starts to sound deliberate.

Of course, industrial accidents are nothing unusual. What is capturing peoples' attention is the scope and frequency of fires, crashes, and explosions. According to this link [*https://www.commdiginews.com/politics-2/commentary/are-food-processing-plant-disasters-part-of-biden-global-food-shortage-143520/*], eight massive industrial accidents happened in 2017. In 2018, it was six. In 2019, it was eight. In 2021, it was eleven. But in just the first four months of 2022, there have been at least seventeen events that have specifically destroyed food processing or fertilizer facilities.

It was the Azure Standard fire that jolted me into greater awareness of the suspicious nature of these incidents. When I mentioned that suspicion to my husband, he was inclined to wave it off. "Sometimes a cigar is just a cigar," he said. Then he, too, read articles about the multitude of food processing plants under siege and agreed strange things were afoot.

As if this isn't odd enough, the U.S. rail carrier Union Pacific made an inexplicable decision to cut fertilizer shipments—why specifically fertilizer?—by 20% just ahead of the spring planting season. This was done without any advanced notice, on April 8. Union Pacific's justification is full of weasel words and makes no logical sense. Why are they cutting shipments of a critical component at such a crucial time, when fertilizer prices are already through the roof? (It's been pointed out that Vanguard, BlackRock, and State Street are the top shareholders of Union Pacific.)

Let's say the quiet part out loud, shall we? Are these events accidental or orchestrated? Are we seeing the beginning of weaponizing food in America? Even Tucker Carlson is asking these questions. As one

Twitter user noted, starvation is a great way to control a population. Intentional or not, these industrial accidents will have an impact on America's food availability. That is irrefutable.

When Biden said we'd have food shortages, I didn't lend him much credence. He's a senile puppet who doesn't know what he's saying most of the time. But maybe, for once, the doddering old man whispered the truth about the people pulling his strings. Certainly, his administration is doing everything in its power—from shutting down pipelines to diverting corn into ethanol rather than animal feed—to hamstring farmers and food processors. As Jeff Crouere at Canada Free Press put it, "It seems as if the president and his administration are doing everything possible to exacerbate the impending food shortage instead of solving it."

But if these attacks were orchestrated, there has to be a purpose or goal behind them. Why would anyone deliberately tighten up food supplies and make products scarce? Is this a planned situation to set up a desired future outcome for the people creating the crisis? Who or what would benefit from this?

As always, the default answer is: Follow the money. However, in this case I believe it's a matter of: Follow the power. Consider this definition of the Cloward-Piven strategy: "A political theory ... that advises activists to create radical change by crashing the system. It encourages the orchestration of various crises designed to push society to the breaking point and steer the populace into embracing an authoritarian socialist government." Make of this what you will.

If you go down the rabbit hole of conspiracy theories, you'll find people speculating that food will soon be government-controlled. Henry Kissinger's famous line is usually quoted: "Who controls the food supply controls the people; who controls the energy can control whole continents; who controls money can control the world."[11]

— compiled by Lou Caverly

CHAPTER THIRTY-ONE

Portraits of Our Fellow-Americans' Food Facilities Sabotaged?

My Patriot Supply, June 10, 2022, had an article that put a personal face on all American food businesses so essential to us all with this devastating headline: "These Are the 20-plus Food Facilities that Have Burned in 2022." Here is an excerpt:

> 2022 has been ESPECIALLY ACTIVE, with over 20 **fires at food facilities so far**—a much higher figure than average. It's gotten a lot of people wondering—including some of the country's largest media outlets—what the heck is going on?
>
> Here are the food facilities that have been hit so far this year:
>
> 1. **Van Drunen Farms Tuthill Facility, Momence, IL** [*Jan. 2*]
> Seven percent of the 80,000-square-foot Van Drunen Farms freeze-drying facility in Momence, Illinois, was burned and declared a "total loss." The fire started at 6 a.m. and no employees were on site. Van Drunen has plants all over the country, but this is their largest—their "main" facility.
> 2. **Cargill-Nutrena Feed Mill, Lecompte, LA** [*Jan. 13*]
> A fire was reported at around 4 a.m. at the 140,000-ton Cargill-Nutrena livestock and pet-feed mill in Lecompte, Louisiana. A building on the property burned for 12 hours and caused no injuries. The fire was blamed on an explosion.

3. **Oregon Potato Company, Warden, WA** [*Jan. 22*]
An explosion attributed to a faulty boiler destroyed the Oregon Potato Company plant in Warden, Washington. This plant supplies corn and potato chips to much of the Western U.S. This fire occurred around noon. Employees called 9-1-1. Seven employees checked into a nearby hospital. No serious injuries were reported. The blaze was the largest the Umatilla County fire district had seen in a decade.
4. **Winston Weaver Company, Winston-Salem, NC** [*Jan. 31*]
At around 7 p.m. on January 31, 150 firefighters were called to a massive fire at the Winston Weaver Company fertilizer plant in Winston-Salem, North Carolina. The blaze was so large that it was allowed to burn. Everyone within a one-mile radius of the plant was ordered to evacuate for fear that the 5,000 tons of finished fertilizer and 600 tons of ammonium nitrate present in the plant would explode. No injuries or deaths were reported—an especially fortunate outcome considering that just a few years earlier, a very similar type of fire at a Weaver Company facility killed 15 people.
5. **Wisconsin River Meats, Mauston, WI** [*Feb. 3*]
An overnight fire destroyed nearly the entire infrastructure of the Wisconsin River Meats manufacturing plant in Mauston, Wisconsin. Most of the plant was considered a total loss. No livestock or employees were injured. Without a facility, co-owner David Mauer says the company will have to rebuild.
6. **Louis Dreyfus Company, Claypool, IN** [*Feb. 16*]
Around 8 p.m., a baghouse used for filtering dust caught fire at the country's largest soy-processing plant. No employees were injured. At the time of the fire, experts worried that the disruption would slow the production of soybean meal in the U.S.
7. **Bess View Farm, St. Albans, VT** [*Feb 18*]
In the early morning of Friday, February 18, a fire devastated the milk parlor at Bess View Farm. Dairy cows had to be transported to facilities in the surrounding areas for care, interrupting Bess View operations. No injuries were reported.

8. **Shearer>s Foods, Hermiston, OR** [*Feb. 22*]
A Shearer's Foods manufacturing plant (specializing in salty snacks, cookies, and crackers) was set ablaze after a boiler exploded, injuring a handful of the over 230 employees of the facility. Former plant safety manager Stephen Dean expressed surprise that no one died, given the extent of the damage. The building will take 15 to 18 months to rebuild.
9. **Nutrien Ag Solution, Sunnyside, WA** [*Feb. 28*]
A fire at the Nutrien Ag Solution facility in Sunnyside, Washington, was reported at around noon on Monday, February 28. An evacuation order was issued to all buildings located within a half-mile radius of the facility. The fire burned through 1.7 million pounds of sulfur used for fertilizer. No one was injured in the blaze.
10. **Nestle Frozen Foods, Jonesboro, AR** [*Mar. 16*]
A fire that took 24 hours to extinguish broke out in a production cooler at the Nestle plant in Jonesboro, Arkansas. The blaze started at 4:30 p.m. None of the 800 plant employees were injured in the fire. The plant produces frozen foods for the Nestle's Hot Pocket, Stouffer's, Lean Cuisine, DiGiorno, and Tombstone brands. The plant was shut down for an extended period, significantly delaying food production.
11. **Wayne Hoover Farm, Longswamp Township, PA** [*Mar 13*]
Fire erupted at around 5 p.m. at the Wayne Hoover dairy farm in Longswamp Township, Pennsylvania. Animals were transported for care to nearby farms and facilities. A total of 42 cows were displaced, significantly disrupting farm operations. No injuries were reported.
12. **Plainfield Walmart Fulfillment Center, Avon, IN** [*Mar. 16*]
A 1.2-million-square-foot Walmart Fulfillment Center (the size of 20 football fields) burned for multiple days in Avon, Indiana—350 firefighters and 30 fire agencies fought the blaze, which consumed massive stocks of food bound for locations all over the country. According to Walmart CEO Doug McMillon, the loss put a "strain" on the company's supply chain system. The Bureau of Alcohol,

Tobacco, Firearms, and Explosives is still investigating the fire's cause, months later.

13. **Penobscot McCrum Potato Processing, Belfast, ME** [*Mar. 24*]
A plant that produces specialty frozen potato products caught fire at 3 a.m. in Belfast, Maine, according to local officials. It is believed that the fire was started in one of the facility's large "fryolator" machines. Witnesses reported that the building on fire was the administrative office. No employees were injured.
14. **Maricopa Food Pantry, Maricopa, AZ** [*Mar 28*]
A sudden fire broke out at the Maricopa Food Pantry in Maricopa, Arizona. The blaze spread quickly, stoked by trailers full of refrigeration fuel. Fifty thousand pounds of food were lost, which will have a detrimental effect on a community which one resident described as not having "many food banks." No one was hurt in the fire.
15. **Rio Fresh, San Juan, TX** [*Mar. 31*]
An enormous fire overtook an onion-packing facility in San Juan, Texas. These key facilities are part of the largest onion-packing operation in southern Texas. No injuries were reported.
16. **East Conway Beef and Pork, Center Conway, NH** [*Apr. 11*]
On the evening of Monday, April 11, a coalition of first responders in Center Conway, New Hampshire, were called to a massive fire at East Conway Beef and Pork. Despite sixteen hours at the scene, the building burned down to the foundation. Neighbors helped save cattle living at the facility. No one was reported injured.
17. **Gem State Processing Plant, Heyburn, ID** [*Apr. 13*]
At approximately 8 a.m., a single-engine plane registered with Spirit Air crashed into the Gem State Processing Plant in Heyburn, Idaho. The pilot was flying solo and was killed in the crash. No other injuries were reported. Gem State Processing Plant sources 18,000 acres of Idaho potatoes.
18. **Taylor Farms, Salinas, CA** [*Apr. 13*]
On the evening of April 13, just after 7 p.m., a four-alarm fire was reported at the Taylor Farms processing facility in Salinas, California. The facility is a food service production and distribution

operation for wholesale salads and shredded lettuce. Because of the threat of combustion from 35,000 pounds of anhydrous ammonia on site, fire officials evacuated the nearby area. The facility was a total loss. Taylor Farms plans to rebuild and reopen the site by spring 2023. No injuries were reported.

19. **Azure Standard, Dufur, OR** [*Apr. 19*]
Organic food distributor Azure Standard lost its headquarters to a fire on April 19. The cause of the fire is under investigation. Azure Standard CEO David Stelzer stated that the headquarters was a total loss and that the company would have to make adjustments to operations and rebuild. No one was injured in the fire.

20. **Nutrien Ag Solution, Leoti, KS** [*Apr. 19*]
For at least the second time in 2022, a Nutrien Ag fertilizer plant caught fire, this time in the small Kansas town of Leoti. The fire broke out at 3:30 p.m. and residents within a half-mile radius of the plant were evacuated. Fire responders reported that the flames were "isolated to a forklift and non-hazardous chemicals." No injuries were reported.

21. **General Mills, Covington, GA** [*Apr. 21*]
A twin-engine Cessna crashed into a General Mills plant in Covington, Georgia, just outside of Atlanta. The plane came to rest in a remote section of the plant's property where empty trailers are stored. According to police, the plane exploded on impact; a small series of explosions followed the crash as well. Two passengers were killed in the crash.

22. **Perdue Farms, Chesapeake, VA** [*Apr. 30*]
Fire broke out at a Perdue Farms grain processing and storage facility in Virginia around 8 p.m. The blaze was centered around a soybean-processing tank. The fire was contained within an hour. The fire had minimum impact on operations. No injuries were reported.

23. **Rail Car Derailment, Ft. Macleod, Alberta, Canada** [*May 22*]
The derailment of a Canadian Pacific Railway freight train in southern Alberta resulted in the loss of 43 rail cars containing potash,

a vital fertilizer ingredient. Some of the cargo was recovered. No injuries were reported. The cause of the derailment is still being investigated.

24. **Forsman Farms, Stockholm Township, MN** [*May 28*]
A massive fire in a small Minnesota township, about an hour west of Minneapolis, killed 200,000 chickens. The fire started around 10 p.m. on May 28 at Forsman Farms. A barn housing many thousands of chickens was burned to the ground. Forsman Farms is one of the largest egg producers in the country and sells more than 3 million eggs a day. The cause of the blaze is being investigated. No injuries were reported.

25. **JBS Foods, Green Bay, WI** [*June 7*]
Firefighters responded quickly to a blaze at a JBS Foods meat packing plant in Green Bay, on the evening of June 7. A small fire inside the plant's meat processing area was controlled within fifteen minutes, saving the entire facility. The fire is being blamed on heat from an auger in the processing area. No injuries were reported.

26. **Festive Foods, Belmont, WI** [*June 13*]
On June 13, the Festive Foods frozen pizza plant in Belmont, Wisconsin, caught fire. More than seventy firefighters were called to the scene, hailing from two dozen departments and four counties. Residents within a mile radius of the plant were advised to keep their windows and doors shut to protect from a dangerous amount of smoke. The fire started "in a compressor room for the refrigeration system while personnel were performing maintenance." No injuries.

The American way of life that holds dear our free enterprise, the worth of the individual and freedom of entrepreneurship must not be lost to NWO hoodlums like "Weathermen-Redux" and "Antifa" types, not while men of Christian faith and courage still exist and firmly retain their guns in America.

— *compiled by Elizabeth Cuppett Caverly*

CHAPTER THIRTY-TWO

Part One: Destruction of Food, Life, and the Planet Itself

THE GREAT BURNING—400 FIRES IN CANADA!

(Lou Caverly, Radio Monologue, June 15, 2023)

One day last week, noticing the strangely hazy morning, I turned on the TV. At once I learned the smoke was not local. In fact, it was not even national. No, four hundred wildfires in Canada had produced vast amounts of smoke that were being carried by the winds down into the northeastern United States. Are the fires a part of God's judgment on Canada and the United States for drifting far, far away from Him? Consider the words of the prophet Joel (chapter 2, verses 1–3):

> Blow ye the trumpet in Zion, and sound an alarm in my holy mountain: let all the inhabitants of the land tremble: for the day of the Lord cometh, for it is nigh at hand; A day of darkness and of gloominess, a day of clouds and of thick darkness, as the morning spread upon the mountains: a great people and a strong; there hath not been ever the like, neither shall be any more after it, even to the years of many generations. A fire devoureth before them; and behind them a flame burneth: the land is as the garden of Eden before them, and behind them a desolate wilderness; yea, and nothing shall escape them.

Though perhaps not at the biblical climactic endpoint of Joel, still this harmful situation suggests God's possible judgment on Canada, a nation that very recently passed legislation facilitating Canadian people to commit assisted suicide!

Physical repercussions of the massive smoke plumes were widespread. Air traffic in several U.S. metro areas was delayed or cancelled. All flights to LaGuardia Airport in New York City were grounded. On Thursday morning more than a thousand flights across the eastern United States were postponed or eliminated. KYW-TV reported that a number of Philadelphia residents called 9-1-1, thinking that some nearby landmark was on fire. In New York Harbor, the Statue of Liberty was quickly engulfed by smog and barely visible. It is ironic for several reasons that this famous American landmark was blacked out. The naive masses believe Lady Liberty represents freedom in a godly-based nation. However, the elite know that French Illuminati Freemasonic groups gave it to America. As such, it is an idol, perhaps being obscured by God's judgment in these four hundred fires. Also, at one point the smoke could be seen from the international space station. The covert occult aspects of agencies like NASA and the 1969 "moon walk narrative" reality—lies and arrogance seem to mark the U.S. space story. All this hubris blasphemes the real ruler of space—God.

Particulate matter in the smoke caused air quality over a wide area to be "extremely hazardous." Health departments warned residents to stay inside if they belonged to any vulnerable categories. One Broadway star, Jodie Comer, was forced to cancel her matinee appearance after struggling to breathe onstage. TV footage at Yankee Stadium showed a thick cloud of orange-brown haze enveloping it. New York streets were also engulfed by this smog.

As school districts in New York and New Jersey announced closures, Windsor Township, seventy miles west of Philadelphia, was perhaps the worst with a particulate matter rating of 457. This compared with a 316 in Delhi, India. How bad was this? Well, India often has the world's most hazardous air quality. Strangely, days after Philadelphia residents called 9-1-1, thinking a major fire was in their city, a real fire crisis developed. A tanker truck caught fire and caused part of a road to collapse, resulting in Route I-95's closure in both directions. More than 26,000 Canadian residents were under evacuation orders as of Thursday, June 8. The fires had already burned more than nine million acres. Government officials, as might be expected, blamed the Canadian fires on hot, dry conditions due to "climate change." (They predicted ongoing drought and long-range global warming.) Is that really the truth? Or are things more ominous?

Satellite images have created suspicions about the real cause of the fires. The *Gateway Pundit* reported that "satellite imagery shared by Wide Awake Media on Twitter shows plumes of smoke rising from at least 17 separate sites [!] ... around 6 p.m. EST. At the 47 second mark ... you can see the smoke stacks begin to emerge almost simultaneously from central and southeast Quebec." *Seventeen simultaneously?* Any possible lightning strikes in the area at the time would be random. These would not hit all at once.

People's Party of Canada leader Maxime Bernier tweeted, "Several arsonists have been arrested in the past weeks in different provinces for lighting forest fires." During the past few months, arsonists have been charged with lighting fires in Nova Scotia, British Columbia, and Alberta. *LifeSite News* reports, "One Albertan, John Cook, has been arrested and charged with 10 counts of arson after setting a string of wildfires in and around Cold Lake, a hamlet near Edmonton."

Perhaps there is a central directive for "Weathermen" saboteurs to accomplish WEF and UN "climate goals" by destroying thousands of cattle and chickens, blowing up thousands of food production facilities in the last year or so, and possibly instigating these latest fires. As an interesting note, when my co-host, Elizabeth, and I broadcast an old Obama-years-era Tom DeWeese article on the original Weathermen radical bombers (many now "respectably" installed in academia and business) we received a sudden influx of NWO intimidation. Were we right over the target—a plan that never quit?

The climate change theory is also challenged by other evidence: Randy DeSoto in *The Western Journal* states, "Quebec is not experiencing a drought, according to the University of Nebraska, Lincoln's North American drought monitor. In fact, just a very small portion of the province has even abnormally dry conditions." Yet the Canadian Interagency Forest Fire Centre showed many of the out-of-control fires were in Quebec. In Quebec City on Thursday the afternoon temperature was only 56 degrees Fahrenheit. It was raining and more rain was on the way. (Hardly the conditions to feed forest fires!) In summation, a small number of arsonists might set a series of wildfires, but they would not do them all at once. That would seem to corroborate that some hugely powerful organized group set the fires in accordance with a carefully laid plan

If so, who are these saboteurs? My colleague, Elizabeth, thinks, "Yes, 'Weathermen, Redux.' This is the global environmental police state control group that includes the World Economic Forum, Pope Francis, John Kerry, King Charles, Justin Trudeau, Joe Biden, and many more of our spiritual and political leaders. Farmland is being torched. Weather wars are producing drought. Starvation and subjugation may soon be coming."

Biblical precedent shows God at times allowing growing chaos to be part of His judgment on people and nations that defy Him and commit abominations. Consider these instances from the Bible:

» Due to his disobedience, Saul would die in battle and his son would not succeed him as king. "And Samuel said unto him, The LORD hath rent the kingdom of Israel from thee this day, and hath given it to a neighbour of thine, that is better than thou" (1 Samuel 15:28).
» Solomon also drifted away from God and worshipped idols: "And Solomon did evil in the sight of the LORD, and went not full after the LORD, as did David his father. Then did Solomon build an high place for Chemosh, the abomination of Moab ... and for Molech, the abomination of the children of Ammon ... Wherefore the LORD said unto Solomon ... I will surely rend the kingdom from thee, and will give it to thy servant" (1 Kings 11: 6–7, 11).
» The nations of Israel and Judah sinned in many ways against God: They worshipped idols; they set up images in the high places and

groves; they sacrificed their children to Molech; they refused to heed the warnings of the prophets. "The Lord removed Israel out of his sight, as he had said by all his servants the prophets. So was Israel carried away out of their own land to Assyria unto this day" (2 Kings 17:23).

» The nation of Judah (the two southern tribes) was also punished for such sins by its defeat at the hands of Nebuchadnezzar, the king of Babylon. "Yet ye have not hearkened unto me, saith the Lord; that ye might provoke me to anger with the works of your own hands to your own hurt ... And this whole land shall be a desolation, and an astonishment; and these nations shall serve the king of Babylon seventy years" (Jeremiah 25:7, 11).

Canada, with new legislation facilitating increased numbers of assisted suicides, and America with its many hospitals doing gender mutilation surgery on young children, are now abominations to God. The two nations have utterly turned away from their Creator

Most people will not repent. Instead, they throw coins, as if before royalty, at "drag queens" doing "the split" in front of innocent children and grandchildren on Memorial Day (Caroline County, Maryland). Immorality abounds. Christian clergy will not repent, either. Like tools of Satan, even famous religious figures like Pope Francis, Albert Mohler, and Franklin Graham advised their Christian congregations to get injected with the COVID mRNA "gene shot." Hence, questionable "vaccines" are still being forced upon the populace. A new "vaccine" called Arexby (SmithGlaxoKline) for the so-called *children's pandemic threat* syncytial respiratory virus (RSV) is being promoted. Strangely, Arexby's *Good Housekeeping* magazine (June 2023) ad is targeted to old people. "Useless Eater" eugenics goals will probably continue to be attained. Disgracefully, *Gain of Function research has not ended!* Sold-out, lying Congress does *nothing* to stop it!

Is God's wrath being kindled against key present-day nations? The great burning of 2023 may well be more than arson or a natural phenomenon. It may be a final warning from Almighty God.

Radio Headline Alert ... Lou Caverly
Dateline: June 29, 2023

SEQUEL: THE GREAT BURNING—500 FIRES!

A hundred new fires in Canada! Twenty-five more in one day! The dangerous smoke is back, with Code Red warnings all over America!

AWFUL AUGUST ALERT
Radio Headline Update ... Lou and Elizabeth Caverly
Dateline: August 10, 2023

THE GREAT BURNING IS BACK—FIRE ERUPTS IN HAWAII!

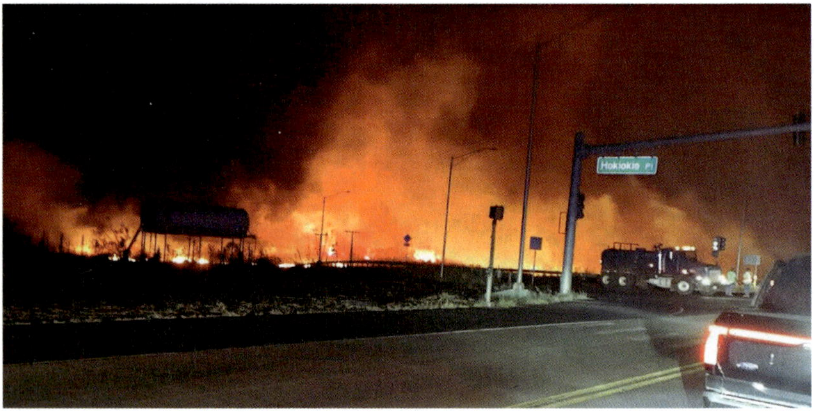

Elizabeth: Danger inside our homes from toxic LED lights, for the Biden Administration has outlawed venerable and beneficial incandescent bulbs. Danger outside with more strange light and fire emerging suspiciously and rapidly in Hawaii.

Lou: August 10, Reuters reports that more than 36 people are dead from wildfires that have swept the island of Maui, Hawaii. It is an "unprecedented disaster." At least 2,100 people have been displaced and many homes and businesses have been destroyed.

The BBC tells that the historic town of Lahaina has burned to the ground—practically nothing is left. The BBC quotes one Lahaina resident as saying, "Every boat in the town harbour is burning."

Hospitals have been overwhelmed by burn and smoke inhalation victims. Thousands have fled from the spreading fires. Some have been running out into the ocean to escape the flames. At least 2,100 people have been displaced and many homes and businesses have been completely destroyed. More than 13,000 homes are without power.

The flames have been fanned by winds from category four Hurricane Dora, which tracked to the west of Maui. Winds have been clocked at over 60 mph. About 4,000 visitors to the popular vacation spot are trying to leave the island. According to the *New York Times*, Kahului Airport remained open, and was sheltering about 1,800 travelers. It also stated, "Non-essential air travel is being discouraged." One Maui resident, Tiere Lawrence, told *Hawaii News Now,* "I don't know where my little brother is ... I don't know where my stepdad is ..."

Once again, the frequency and intensity of these fires seem highly suspicious. Are they all due to natural causes? We can't help but think there is a very high probability that devious forces in league with Satan are responsible.

Elizabeth: You're the mathematician, Lou, who can compute probabilities. Yet, it's becoming crystal clear to ***all of us, an NWO sabotage pattern is killing*** thousands of pigs, chickens, cattle, and exploding or burning hundreds of food production facilities. Raging fires are being used to destroying land and our future crops worldwide.

CHAPTER THIRTY-THREE

Part 2: Destruction of Food, Life, and the Planet Itself

EARTH UNDER SIEGE I: COMING CATACLYSM MUST BE CURTAILED

(Lou Caverly ... Radio Monologue ... Sept. 5, 2022)

Health Ranger Mike Adams recently interviewed Dane Wigington of GeoengineeringWatch.org. Adams summarized the content of the interview at NaturalNews.com, September 2, 2022:

> The entire planet is being deliberately plunged into a global famine nightmare, achieved via geoengineering programs carried out by world governments trying to achieve global depopulation.
>
> That's the warning from Dane Wigington of Geoengineering-Watch.org, a site dedicated to the scientific investigation of the global "kill switch" portfolio of technologies being used to control weather and cause the collapse of the world's life-sustaining biosphere.
>
> The simultaneous droughts, floods, and freak weather events we are observing right now across the globe are not natural weather events, Wigington warns. They are "engineered" weapons being deployed against humanity under the cover of blaming "climate change."
>
> In today's Situation Update podcast, we feature a full one-hour interview with Dane Wigington, where we delve into the multiple vectors of a global attack on the food supply, the biosphere, phytoplankton in aquatic ecosystems, and life as we know it on planet Earth.

Adams' list of major shocks discussed with Dane Wigington:

1. Detailed discussions of atmospheric alterations to attack the biosphere of Earth
2. How weather weapons are used to cause mass famine and starvation across the planet
3. How atmospheric spraying is altering soil pH and obliterating forests and crops
4. Discussion around "The Dimming" and chemtrails and their true purpose
5. Why BILLIONS of humans will die if we don't stop the planetary genocide soon

My Divided Kingdom Radio co-anchor (and mate), Elizabeth Cuppett Caverly and I were beyond shocked by one-man-hero Dane Wigington's well-documented, draconian warning. I felt it essential to listen to the interview again more closely and extract my own list of points. It is clear that there is a continuing blasting of the ionosphere, punching holes in it—a concern discussed in Elizabeth's 2004 book, *Patriot's Warning II: Chaos and Chemtrails.*

Now, against the backdrop of the COVID-19 vaccine depopulation scenario, these earlier DVDs, "What in the World Are They Spraying?" and "Why in the World Are They Spraying?" are once again relevant. The pH of the soil is being altered, not in a good way for humans to live.

This insane ionosphere blasting with HAARP *et al.* is destroying the ozone layer at unprecedented levels. When you go outside, your DNA (animals' and plants', too) is being damaged! Now, without ozone protection, UVC rays that never before reached your skin are striking your body. Possibly even X-rays can now reach through the broken ozone protection layer. These, in fact, represent an assault on all human, animal, and plant life on Earth ... Yes, where are the bees? ...

More deadly details from the September 2 interview:

- » World governments look upon weather as weapons of war, sometimes used against their own people.

- Even mainstream media finally admits weather modification is real.
- Not only is the DNA of plants, animals, and humans being damaged, but plankton populations are down as much as 90 percent, jeopardizing the entire ocean ecosystem, as well as reducing oxygen in the atmosphere.
- Storms, including hurricanes, are being stalled or guided to particular target cities or states by use of microwaves from both land- and sea-based radar.
- Heating of the ionosphere by devices like HAARP can create a "high-pressure heat dome" that blocks rain and leads to higher temperatures.
- Such methods are being used to direct rain north into Canada and Alaska, and then eventually down on the East Coast. So, the West has extreme drought, but not the East. [Adams and Wigington believe the East is left till last to be harmed in order to dupe them until the end stages of this depopulation scenario.]
- Spraying with particulate matter such as aluminum and barium can increase the pH of soil. Excessive particles lead to large cloud formations, but no rain. The makers of the film "Why in the World Are They Spraying" documented this well—how eventually crops would not thrive or even grow. Planned eventual worldwide famine?
- Aluminum in spraying is especially harmful even if it falls on acid soil. It kills off plants and beneficial soil bacteria. Dane, who left one whole life's work to devote himself to warning the world of this coming disaster, remarks darkly, "The soil microbiome is done."
- People are lulled into complacency by governments. They have the attitude, "The leaders wouldn't do that to themselves." But they would and do, even if they, too, will be the victims, Adams and Wigington conclude.

As a mathematician and watchman-journalist, I, Lou Caverly, would have to agree their plan is, in essence, committing (their own) suicide. WE MUST STOP THIS!

EARTH UNDER SIEGE II: LESSER DEATH BY DUMBNESS

(Lou Caverly ... Radio Monologue ... Sept. 5, 2022)

The September 2 interview at Brighteon.com between Mike Adams and Dane Wigington also discussed the topic of "renewable energy." Mike Adams quipped, "Green energy only works if you don't use it." He elaborated:

> Did you know that Amazon fulfillment centers are catching on fire due to solar panel installation on their roofs? It turns out all that "green" energy is a fire hazard. Remarkably, as CNBC.com reports, 12.7% of Amazon's buildings that feature solar installations have caught fire due to "arcing" from the solar installations.
>
> It looks like "going green" also means going up in flames.
>
> If you were a business owner and saw that a new energy system was setting fire to 12.7% of your warehouses, you would shut it down. That's exactly what Amazon did, too.
>
> So, when the sun is shining, solar power is catching buildings on fire. When the sun isn't shining, solar produces zero energy.
>
> Remember, too, that you're supposed to buy an electric vehicle but not charge it, because charging it might collapse the power grid in California, utility officials have warned.
>
> So green energy only works when you don't use it.

Dane and Mike then debunked the validity of much of the "climate change" agenda:

- » The expense of replacing batteries in an electric vehicle. The batteries can only be charged a limited number of times. Replacing them can cost over $10,000.
- » Lithium batteries present a fire hazard. They also present an environmental hazard in mining the lithium and in the disposal of old batteries.

» At the present time, there are not nearly enough charging stations. A huge investment in station infrastructure and power generation facilities will be needed to make electric vehicles a viable alternative to present transportation.
» None of the alternative sources of electric energy—wind, solar, hydroelectric—are reliable, especially given the damage done by [sky] geoengineering.
» The high cost of electricity makes it difficult to grow food plants indoors, especially on a large scale. This will contribute to food shortages.
» Dane highly recommends the film "Planet of the Humans," which explains how non-renewable so-called "renewable energy" really is.

[Also, check out the video, "The Dimming," at GeoengineeringWatch.org.]

Only the dimwitted can extol wind farms that kill bald eagles, but do not run when there is no breeze. Then, too, there are more dummies who don't even comprehend that fossil fuel coal is essential to make electricity for the much-vaunted electric cars. I close with a few chuckles from one of our listeners. He reported his town gave local approval to build charging stations in front of McDonalds. Good luck to California if it thinks it can mandate only electric cars statewide by 2035.

EXTINCTION PROTOCOLS ALERT—BEYOND EMERGENCY

(Lou Caverly ... Radio Monologue ... July 12, 2023)

Elizabeth and I were trying to find some R&R on the weekend after the Fourth. It seemed there was no sun, only persistent chemtrails. I noticed that climate watchman Dane Wiggington had a new July 6 interview with Health Ranger Mike Adams. Any of you who did not read my two essays on Dane's warnings should visit our website, DividedKingdomRadio.com, and look under "Breaking News" for my two radio monologues listed under September 5, 2022.

As Elizabeth and all of you know, I am not an alarmist. I am a mathematician and a usually calm guy from the Northeast, with a somewhat JFK-like accent. So, when the new Dane Wiggington interview of July 6 was concluded and Elizabeth asked me my opinion, she really opened her eyes wide. Instead of my usual understatement, I said these words: "If Dane is correct, this could be the end of all humanity. In fact, of all life on earth."

We must get the word out everywhere. We are counting on all of you. Even the sanest members of the high elite must be shocked into STOPPING THIS "GEOENGINEERING" that now Biden [*Daily Mail*, July 1] announces out in the open (even though Dane says weather modification has been going on for seventy-five years).

CIRCULATE THESE BULLET POINTS OUT TO EVERYONE YOU KNOW! In addition to the delineation of planetary harm I covered in my first two essays, here are the latest Dane Wiggington exposés, warnings, and stats:

» Life support systems are being destroyed forever. (The plankton layer in the ocean is 90 percent gone.)
» The ozone layer is being annihilated. This will cause many increased cancers in humans.
» This geoengineering, microwaving done ostensibly to disintegrate methane, brings only a temporary cooling effect. Wiggington reveals that (black project?) (Project Alamo and possibly others) are going on. Hidden chambers in cell towers are being used to beam these microwaves into the ionosphere.
» Chemical ice nucleation is resulting in baseball-sized hail—certainly harmful to crops. Dane discussed one location that had a temperature of 30 degrees, but some of this synthetic snow/ice that had been on the ground for two days had a temperature of only 15 degrees! At our own home in the recent days of heavy chemtrailing, we suddenly had a hail storm.
» When I edited Elizabeth Cuppett Caverly's 2004 book, *Patriot's Warning II: Chaos and Chemtrails*, it was noted that labs had detected aluminum and barium from chemtrails even in some

streams. Now, Dane Wiggington reports the following extremely toxic components are in the sprayed chemtrail mix: manganese, ***strontium,*** aluminum, barium, graphene, and polymer fibers. The latter can carry any desired biological weapons. Elizabeth's book mentioned microplasmic fungi spores.

» Is this part of the depopulation agenda? Aluminum, states Wiggington (former forestry worker and expert), will kill the root, preventing nutrients from going into the plant. Fifteen years ago, he states, the success rate for saplings planted was 95 percent. Now the rate for new saplings to live one year is 0 percent!
» "We're in a kill zone," commented Health Ranger Mike Adams (NaturalNews.com). "Humans have been labeled for extinction. I think they'll kill 1–2 billion before ending this. Famine will do it, too"
» Wiggington agreed, expanding on the role of wildfires in this famine scenario, "Since May 1, on average, we're losing 330,000 acres every day, with a total of 20 million acres and counting."
» Wiggington asserted that the globalist goal has "each country taking its turn," so that, he says, "even in Siberia, acres are burning, too." [We wonder if that kind of reciprocal cooperation among countries is used in the worldwide destruction of chickens, cows, food manufacturing facilities, and petroleum refineries, and now, raging radical Islamic chaos, presently occurring in France.]
» A military document is titled, "Forest fires are a military weapon." "This could be indicative," Wiggington says, "that there was real preparation ahead of time for two or more of these fires."
» Fir trees are in massive die-off in the western U.S.A.
» "The Dimming," ***A MUST-SEE*** video at GeoengineeringWatch.org shows how this diabolical geoengineering BLOCKS ESSENTIAL PHOTOSYNTHESIS. At 104 degrees Fahrenheit, photosynthesis stops! So, heating up the ionosphere is far from good.
» Nature has produced 75 percent of the world's gross domestic product (GDP). So besides causing famine and death, "dimming"

can devastate the world's economy, too.

- 60 million tons of nanoparticles a year are being put in the air. Dane says, "At the Paradise Fire, there was a documented blanket of aerosol spraying on top of the smoke layer, so whatever that's about, it's not benevolent."
- Necessary to all of us, honey bee pollinators, are being vitiated by aluminum. They're packed full of it. They get Alzheimer's and can't even fly straight to get to their hive. The numbers of honeybees had already been shown to be greatly decimated over the last years. Now even that number is down another 48 percent!
- Psychopathic leaders have no realization they are harming even themselves in doing things like dumping half a million barrels of DDT off the LA coast. (This synergistically escalates the effects of other toxins, like aluminum and mercury, by 10,000 percent.) Some demented climate engineering gurus are even proposing nuclear devices launched from ships in the South Seas. Like kids without a clue playing a video game—this is how murderously insane this blindness to reason is ... We are all sane. If we remain quiet and do not end this (calling on leaders in high places, too) we are ensuring our own eventual suicide.

Dean Wiggington states, "If we don't stop this now, none of us will be here. It will take all of us. If you die, taking your last breath, *doing right*, it will be all right." This is Lou speaking. God commands every one of you reading or hearing this to tell a person or many persons. **THIS IS AN EXTINCTION ALERT.**

CHAPTER THIRTY-FOUR

Evil Oracles Materializing?

"Emergency Alert: FDA Approves Anthrax 'Vaccine' as Biden Creates New Permanent Office of Pandemic Preparedness and Response Policy"

(Elizabeth Cuppett Caverly ... Radio Monologue ... August 3, 2023) On our Divided Kingdom Radio broadcast, Thursday evening, July 27, we quoted a masterful essay by Frank Wright, LifeSite News, March 30, 2023: "The Real enemy is humanity itself; exposing The Club of Rome's climate agenda." In this excellent article, Wright documented the immense influence globalist and New Age occultist Maurice Strong had on the environmental movement, both in the U.N. and as head of the World Economic Forum.

Unbelievably, twenty-three years ago, "guru" Strong (led probably by the same Theosophist "ascended masters" Alice Bailey claimed guided her) was an amazing augur of the COVID-shot catastrophe and the aftermath we are facing. Some credible sources estimate the Earth's population, consequently, has suddenly gone from about 7 billion down to 5 billion people. Frank Wright tells us about Maurice Strong's uncanny prediction: "In his autobiography, ***Where on Earth Are We Going,*** *Strong projected that* ***in 2031, 'the human tragedy would be on a scale hitherto unimagined.'" He also wrote that the brightest prospect lay in forecasts that two-thirds of the world's already diminished population might be wiped out.*** WEF head Klaus Schwab (who recruited Maurice Strong earlier to lead the WEF) has recently reiterated a less homicidal echo of Strong's grisly prediction. Klaus Schwab says that by 2031 you'll have nothing and be happy about it.

Habakkuk 2:2 instructs God's watchmen to write warnings on tablets so that **"The people can run ..."** This warning aspect/obligation of the Divided Kingdom radio program is a key component of why we believe God called us to first go on air in fall 2003. A "Red Flag" warning has just come into view. It is a little more than a year until 2025, a Bill Gates "target" year. Is more trouble, indeed, ahead, akin to the COVID-era scourge? Globalist Bill Gates has openly stated that Earth's people can look for a new pandemic—possibly one to target children badly—in the year 2025. Already, Gates' Foundation and Johns Hopkins University have held 2025 preparatory drills.

The World Health Organization (WHO), possibly the key enforcer of a future pharma-medical police state, was not able in 2023 to get nations of the world to ratify its pandemic treaty. Prayers of many persons were answered the year before, also, when many prayed and called Congress, opposing the U.S. adoption of draconian WHO pandemic amendments. Next year the treaty will again be pushed (with our great surveillance and protests needed at that time). No one wants a new world of forced injections and quarantine prison camps.

(In Scripture, I believe God may have given me a "word of knowledge" recently. It is that His people "have about one year" in which to prepare quickly.) Note: it is a little more than a year until 2025, the Bill Gates "target" year. Reinforcing this danger warning, two concerning news items have suddenly appeared in July 2023. Interestingly, we were just compiling the news articles for tonight's program when another amazing anthrax article came in the mail from our friend, Brother Bruce. This seemed heaven-sent to help us put the two jigsaw puzzle pieces together ...

First, the *Gateway Pundit*'s July 25 headline states: ***"Biden Creates New 'Permanent Office of Pandemic Preparedness and Response Policy,' Laying Foundation for Medical Martial Law."*** According to GP's guest writer, Leo Hohman, a ***military*** man, retired Air Force Major General Paul Friedrichs has been appointed by Joe Biden to head this new ***permanent*** office. The writer points out that the precedent for putting America under military control was certainly set in motion by "Operation Warp Speed." [See how a military-medical police state template is being set up, ***permanently***.]

A second article is very worrisome, too. This alerting article was from The People's Voice.tv, July 24. Headline: ***"FDA Approves 'Experimental Anthrax Vaccine' for All U.S. Citizens."*** *Emergent BioSolutions, the vaccine maker, has received FDA approval for all adults aged 18-65. The article states, "The controversial vaccine, Cyfendus, is approved for use despite having only been tested on animals, according to Reuters."*

[We have noted that Big Pharma drugs sometimes seem to hold a hidden depopulation message in their nomenclature. For instance: Prevagen ["Prev" = Prevent and "gen" = genes. Is the hidden meme "Prevent genes from working"?]; and now we come to Cyfendus—sounds a lot like "Defend us," doesn't it? ["Cy" can be short for "cyto," referring to "cells." Could "fend" mean "fend off"?] Will the hapless cells of the body have to fend off still another depopulation agent? Remember how top researchers have shown COVID spike proteins get into and transform humanity's original God-given DNA.

Our oblivion to coming trouble is what globalists count on. They want sleeping, "Bread and Circus" people. ***Nothing gets in the way of the progress of a soon-coming world military-medical police state.*** *Recall how the Department of Defense (DoD) implemented the anthrax mandate for U.S. military personnel in 1998. Service members' reports of extreme adverse effects finally led to congressional hearings in early 2000. The U.S. House of Representatives Committee on Government Reform recommended halting the mandatory program,* ***although it was not officially halted.***

Be warned. Prepare, without delay.

Postscript: August 1, 2023—More vital info about the FDA approved anthrax vaccine coming up. In this Natural News excerpt, Olivia Cook writes the following important warnings:

FDA approves ANTHRAX vaccine despite its TOXIC INGREDIENTS

Cyfendus has only been tested in animal models of inhalation anthrax.

However, Emergent said a Phase 2 clinical study has shown its non-interference with antibacterial drugs. A Phase 3 trial that measured its lot consistency, immunogenicity, and safety following a two-dose schedule yielded successful results. (Related: FDA uses 'animal' rule to approve anthrax vaccine for humans. ... You're just an experimental animal to the vaccine industry.)

But the product's package insert revealed the dangerous ingredients in every vial of Cyfendus. The insert disclosed that the anthrax shot uses two adjuvants, one with aluminum and the new synthetic adjuvant CPG7909. It also contains a saline solution containing formaldehyde and benzethonium chloride as preservatives.

Commonly used as an adjuvant in vaccines, aluminum is a known cytotoxin and neurotoxin. Formaldehyde has been branded as "carcinogenic to humans" by the World Health Organization's International Agency for Research on Cancer (IARC) based on sufficient evidence it can cause nasopharyngeal cancer and leukemia.

Meanwhile, benzethonium chloride—an ammonium compound often found in detergents—has been found to be irritating and harmful to mucous membranes at concentrations as low as one percent. Higher concentrations of this chemical are highly toxic if ingested.

Dr. Meryl Nass, an expert on bioterrorism and anthrax expounded on her skepticism in a Substack article, noting that the FDA itself has admitted it does not work. Nass said the vaccine requires antibiotics alongside it, "and it is the antibiotics that actually kill anthrax after an acute exposure."

"You can't be sprayed with anthrax, get vaccinated and then patiently wait a month to develop immunity—you'd be dead by then. Plus, if you lived—you would, of course, show immunity by a month because you were just exposed to anthrax."

Nass also cited that BioThrax, the predecessor of Cyfendus, "caused birth defects." An observational study on the anthrax shot found that "there were more birth defects in infants born to individuals vaccinated with BioThrax in the first trimester, compared to individuals vaccinated post pregnancy or individuals never vaccinated."

> "This shot [Cyfendus] is the old anthrax shot with a novel adjuvant added—so it cannot possibly be safer than the bad old vaccine," the expert continued. She also mentioned the "horrendous" effects of the injection—with 84 percent of trial participants experiencing a systemic reaction and 64 percent having limited use of the arm the vaccine was injected in.

The importance of the second key warning in my August 3 radio monologue, the setting up of a "Permanent Office of Pandemic Preparedness and Response Policy" using military adjunct control, cannot be emphasized too much.

If the U.S. eventually goes completely under the jurisdiction of the World Health Organization (WHO), when and if the WHO Pandemic Treaty is ratified, then forced pandemic injections and mandatory quarantine camps will likely come to America.

What other dangers lie ahead? **Mike Adams, July 30, 2023 (Natural News)** *has a very grave twelve-point prognostication* that we excerpt here:

> **TWELVE UNDENIABLE SIGNS GLOBALISTS ARE ENGINEERING THE END OF HUMANITY**
>
> It's no longer taboo to publicly talk about *depopulation*. Even many who once dismissed the concept as a *conspiracy theory* are now publicly acknowledging the reality that global efforts are underway to drastically reduce the human population on planet Earth.
>
> Mainstream media now frequently talks about "climate lockdowns" as a good thing—to cease human activity on planet Earth in order to "save the planet" from so-called *climate change*, a wholesale fabrication and fake science fraud rooted in the lie that carbon dioxide is somehow bad for life on the planet. (Without it, there would be no photosynthesis, no plants, no animals, and no humans.)
>
> Now, corporate media is openly calling for climate blackouts and lockdowns, the rationing of air conditioning and possibly even banning the use of electricity to cool homes and buildings during hot weather days. This is all being positioned as necessary to save

the planet, of course. The *Los Angeles Times*, for example, recently published a story asking whether an "occasional blackout" might "help solve climate change."

As Slay News has correctly pointed out:

Green agenda alarmists in the corporate media are now calling for widespread electrical grid blackouts for "the greater good" of "solving the climate crisis." In an article from the Los Angeles Times, *the establishment media outlet argues that it would be "easier and less expensive to fight climate change" if the public would "be willing to live with" blackouts.*

We are past the point, in other words, of the controlled corporate media saying that engineered blackouts and climate lockdowns are just a conspiracy theory. Now, the controlled media is openly claiming that ***the functioning of human society will destroy the planet*** [emphasis added]. Therefore, they imply, the only way to save the planet is to take down the food and energy infrastructure that keeps humanity alive.

The current population of human beings on planet Earth, of course, is a function of affordable food powered by affordable, abundant energy (mostly in the form of fossil fuels). Ending this—which is now the admitted goal of climate cultists, Democrats, and the same "science" community that told us COVID vaccines were safe and effective—will inevitably result in global depopulation of the human race. No fuel = no farms. No farms = no food. No food = no people. This is the openly admitted goal.

Here, I list twelve undeniable signs that globalists are actively seeking the extermination of the human race from this planet. Note that all twelve of these signs are readily verifiable.

#1) **They are terraforming the planet through planetary-scale atmospheric alterations**—Large-scale efforts are underway right now to alter the chemistry of planet Earth in order to make it inhospitable to human life by removing CO_2 from the atmosphere through "carbon sequestration" efforts. Since CO_2 is necessary for all photosynthesis—which drives the web of life on planet Earth—this effort would collapse all food crops, rainforests, marine ecosystems, and more, ultimately killing off virtually all animals and human beings on the planet if not stopped.

2) **The biometric inventory of the human race (WorldCoin) has begun, and all humans will be "inventoried" so that globalists can properly track their depopulation milestones**—The WorldCoin effort to scan everyone's eyeballs and create an encryption key based on their biometrics is actually a "human inventory" scheme to digitally record all the human beings known to exist on the planet. This step is necessary to track human depopulation milestones and identify anyone who has not been inventoried by the system ...

3) **They've given up on educating young people to be prepared for a productive future**—Notice that government-run schools no longer teach anything resembling practical skills, independent thinking, or even basic knowledge needed to carry out jobs in a productive society. This is because there is no plan to deploy the younger generations of human beings in any productive activity whatsoever. The plan is to exterminate them.

4) **Controlled demolition of energy infrastructure that drives human economies**—As discussed above, the planned take-down of the energy infrastructure is engineered to cause both economic collapse and food scarcity leading to mass starvation.

5) **Governments are funding, developing, and deploying anti-human genetic bioweapons**—As if engineered starvation and economic collapse weren't enough by themselves, Western governments like the United States of America are continuing to fund genetic bioweapons that target the human race. The *spike protein* is one such weapon, and it was engineered into both the COVID *plandemic* and the mRNA vaccines which are designed to maim and kill as many human beings as possible. The U.S. Dept. of Defense is the instigator of these bioweapons, and they have a long history of running illegal bioweapons laboratories in countries like Ukraine (and various African nations as well) while actively developing *self-replicating bioweapons* which feature ethnic targeting based on genetic differences in biology.

6) **There is a coordinated, global effort to destroy seed**

diversity and make crops unable to reproduce—To make sure that free people can't grow their own food, a global effort is also under way to control the seed supply and to collapse seed diversity while transitioning agriculture to toxic, genetically-engineered seeds that grow crops which synthesize pesticide chemicals right into the crop itself (such as with GM corn). Seed giants like Monsanto (now Bayer) have bought up many smaller seed suppliers over the years, wiping out seed diversity. This centralization in the hands of a few, powerful corporations is one of the necessary steps to **weaponizing food scarcity** and using engineered famine.

7) **Rapid rollout of automation robots to replace blue collar workers and transport drivers**—Warehouse workers will soon be replaced by bipedal warehouse robots that can handle nearly all the same tasks.

8) **Rise of AI systems to replace white-collar workers: Journalists, artists, coders, writers, and more**—Regenerative AI systems like ChatGPT are on the move and will soon replace journalists, writers, coders, business managers, and much more.

9) **The CDC is rolling out recommendations for annual COVID injections until you die**—According to *The Blaze*, new CDC director, Dr. Mandy Cohen, plans to push for annual COVID shots just like annual flu shots.

10) **Geoengineering-driven global famine to unleash mass starvation**—This point refers to geoengineering weather control that guides water mass dispersion to produce floods, droughts, storms, or anything else that can damage crops and cause widespread food scarcity and food inflation.

11) **Infertility chemicals are being placed in the food supply (atrazine, glyphosate, hormone disruptors) to reduce population sustainability**—It's true that atrazine, the No. 2 most common herbicide in our food supply, is a chemical castrator that "turns the frogs gay." In doing so, it also causes loss of reproductive viability, leading to population reduction. We currently test for atrazine in our mass spec food science laboratory, and we can confirm that we are seeing

atrazine in the human food supply. We also test for glyphosate and heavy metals, among other things, and we see a lot of contamination of the food supply chain.

12) **Globalists are preparing to initiate the end of debt-based economics that have driven cheap food and affordable growth of human populations**—Globalist banks will ditch dollars and call for a global switch to a CBDC system where they can surveil and control all your income sources and expenditures. (Download my new audio book, *Resilient Prepping* at ResilientPrepping.com—it teaches you how to survive the total collapse of civilization and the loss of both the power grid and combustion engines.)

Lou Caverly and I, Elizabeth Cuppett Caverly, co-hosts at Divided Kingdom Radio.com and co-authors of this book, *COVID and Coming Chaos*, want to encourage all readers of this book that, no matter what turmoil and harsh tests may lie ahead, Jesus Christ will be your personal friend and helper. He gives us the power to live an abundant life here on Earth and to live eternally with Him. Miracles can and will happen during times of great tribulation.

Alexander B. Cuppett, the late former action officer to the joint chiefs of staff and religious watchman, recounted the true story of his late nineteenth-century pastor-ancestor, J.C. Skipper, who was being chased by a formidable bear. When J.C. Skipper reached Maryland's Deep Creek Lake, God "translated" him safely and miraculously across the lake.

Even as CBDC (Central Bank Digital Currency) and "Mark of the Beast" may be coming closer, God can and will supernaturally help His true sheep. These are the ones who have separated from the world's evils and put their trust in Jesus and obey God's commandments.

Our book, the one you have just read, is called *COVID and Coming Chaos. Its successor (whether or not it's a real book later, or whether God simply engraves it in your deepest hearts) will honor JESUS, "OUR HOPE IN THE COMING CHAOS." Our love and prayers to all of you!*

—Lou and Elizabeth Caverly

REFERENCES

Chapter 2: ***Clandestine Experimentation: Injury and Death to the Populace***

1. Horowitz, Leonard G., *Emerging Viruses: AIDS and Ebola*, Tetrahedron Publishing, 1997, p. 288
2. Aidsbiowarfare.com
3. Horowitz, p. 275
4. Ibid, p. 309–310
5. Prisonplanet.com, "U.S. keeping secret stash of smallpox viruses at lab in Georgia to use for future bioweapons," June 8, 2011
6. NaturalNews.com, "In Explosive Interview, author of Bioweapons Act Dr. Francis Boyle confirms coronavirus is an 'offensive biological warfare weapon,'" Feb. 4, 2020
7. BigLeaguePolitics.com, "President of World Academy of Biomedical Sciences Says COVID-19 is Bioweapon Created in Wuhan Lab," August 14, 2020

Chapter 27: ***Poison Food***

8. "American Farmers to Inject Livestock with mRNA Shots This Month," Infowars.com, April 7, 2023

Chapter 29: ***Global Food Supply—Sabotage, Control, and Coming Famine***

9. https://d18rnop25nwr6d.cloudfront.net/CIK-0001364742/3173f90f-150e-43a3-941a-fba9a7e35773.pdf

Chapter 30: ***Global Food Supply—Sabotage, Control, and Coming Famine***

10. Tyler Durden, "Food Processing Plant Fires," *Zero Hedge*, April 30, 2022